Marketing Health Behavior

Principles, Techniques, and Applications

Marketing Health Behavior

Principles, Techniques, and Applications

Edited by

LEE W. FREDERIKSEN

Virginia Polytechnic Institute and State University
Blacksburg, Virginia

LAURA J. SOLOMON

University of Vermont
Burlington, Vermont

and

KATHLEEN A. BREHONY

Phobia Clinic of Southwest Virginia
Roanoke, Virginia

PLENUM PRESS • NEW YORK AND LONDON

Library of Congress Cataloging in Publication Data

Main entry under title:

Marketing health behavior.

Includes bibliographical references and index.

1. Preventive health services—Marketing. 2. Health education—Marketing. 3. Marketing—Social aspects. 4. Medicine and psychology. I. Frederiksen, Lee W. II. Solomon, Laura J. III. Brehony, Kathleen A.

RA427.M295 1984 613 84-3271

ISBN 0-306-41523-2

A Division of Plenum Publishing Corporation

233 Spring Street, New York, N.Y. 10013

Printed in the United States of America

Contributors

Kathleen A. Brehony, Phobia Clinic of Southwest Virginia, Roanoke, Virginia

Lee W. Frederiksen, Department of Psychology, Virginia Polytechnic Institute and State University, Blacksburg, Virginia

David Garner, Live for Life Program, Johnson & Johnson, New Brunswick, New Jersey

Philip Kotler, J. L. Kellogg Graduate School of Management, Northwestern University, Evanston, Illinois

John E. Martin, Veterans Administration Medical Center, Jackson, Mississippi

Patrick E. Murphy, Department of Marketing, Marquette University, Milwaukee, Wisconsin

William D. Novelli, Porter, Novelli & Associates, 3240 Prospect Street, NW, Washington, D.C.

Donald M. Prue, Veterans Administration Medical Center, Jackson, Mississippi

Douglas S. Solomon, formerly with the *Stanford Heart Disease Prevention Program,* Stanford University, Stanford, California; currently with Apple Computer, San Jose, California

Laura J. Solomon, Department of Psychology, University of Vermont, Burlington, Vermont

Graham W. Ward, School of Medicine, Tufts University, Boston, Massachusetts

Curtis S. Wilbur, Live for Life Program, Johnson & Johnson, New Brunswick, New Jersey

Preface

This is a book that grew out of frustration. The frustration was rooted in our failed attempts to help people modify health-related behavior. From a behavioral medicine perspective, it was readily apparent to us that there were many things people could do to improve their health. Some of these were preventive behaviors, whereas others were much more therapeutic or rehabilitative in nature. Put another way, there were specific well-known behavioral strategies that people could use to maintain or regain their good health. Yet despite our good intentions, enthusiasm, and considerable efforts, something was wrong. People dropped out of therapy or failed to follow behavioral prescriptions. Workshops and clinics were half-empty. If people would attend workshops or follow therapeutic programs, their health would benefit. Yet in our experience and in the experience of most of our colleagues, compliance to treatment programs was a major problem.

Faced with such a situation, it is easy to blame the victim—in this case the client. It is common to hear therapists talk of poorly motivated clients, complain that people are just not interested in improving their health, or even speculate about people's self-destructive tendencies. Although this may be comforting to the therapist, it does very little to solve the problem. What was needed was an approach to improve adherence to therapeutic programs rather than comforting excuses for their failure. It is in this context that we became exposed to the area of social marketing.

The notion of marketing seems to be a natural for overcoming the problems associated with low adherence to behavioral medicine programs. Could we not apply the same principles used to sell cigarettes, alcohol, and fast foods to the promotion of regular exercise, smoking cessation, and a healthful diet? The notion that principles derived from commercial marketing could be successfully applied to the promotion of desirable behavior had already been developed under the term of *social marketing*.

To some readers, behavioral medicine and social marketing may seem to be strange bedfellows. Behavioral medicine is focused largely on the behavior of the individual and his or her immediate environment. Further, it tends to be clinical in orientation. Behavioral medicine practitioners see themselves as professional health care providers.

On the other hand, social marketing is large scale in focus and methodology. It deals with populations and market segments, not individuals. Social marketing practitioners have varied backgrounds, but their roots are often in commercial marketing. To complicate the integration of social marketing and behavioral medicine further, we have found that for many people within behavioral medicine the very mention of the word *marketing* conjures up images of manipulation, hucksterism, and fast-talking salesmen in plaid pants.

As formidable as these barriers may seem initially, we have found that the integration of social marketing and behavioral medicine is a natural one. Both social marketing and behavioral medicine are fundamentally data-based, systematic approaches to changing behavior. In each case, the approach is one of experimentation—finding what works to alter people's actions. There are also many parallels in the terminology and general approach. In each case for example, one begins with a well-specified objective and a comprehensive assessment of what really exists.

We also found that the benefits of this integration were many. For example, a social marketing perspective inspired us to question many unnoticed assumptions of how programs might be structured, where they might be delivered, and how they might be promoted. Should all programs be delivered once a week in the health care provider's office? What about on-site delivery tailored to the participants' schedules? In short, the marketing perspective emphasizes tailoring the program to the needs of the people to be reached. It replaces frustration and a search for excuses with a specific, systematic, and useful approach to solving the problem of low adherence to programs.

The purpose of this volume is twofold. Part I focuses on outlining the principles and techniques relevant to marketing health behavior. Part II explores the application of these principles to specific health behavior problems.

The first chapter in Part I, which was written by the editors, provides a framework for the remainder of the volume. It explores the development of behavioral medicine and the need for a marketing perspective. It outlines the components of the social marketing approach and suggests how they can be applied to the problems of changing health-related behaviors. Emphasis is placed both on the underlying similarities of the two fields as well as on the unique contribution of the social marketing perspective.

Chapter 2 was written by Philip Kotler, a noted social marketing expert. He describes the roots of social marketing by comparing and contrasting them to those of the other marketing approaches. He also outlines the social marketing process and provides illustrations of how it can be applied to health-related behaviors.

Chapter 3 covers one of the key concepts of social marketing, namely, analyzing markets. It was written by Patrick Murphy, an experienced social marketer and researcher. This chapter highlights the importance of marketing research and the related consideration of market segmentation. It details the variables to be considered in each approach and provides a strategy for relating market research to market segmentation.

Chapter 4's author is William Novelli, one of the most accomplished social marketers in this country. Novelli documents the marketing process and takes the reader through the six critical stages of actually developing marketing programs in the health area. This chapter is the bridge that links marketing concepts to how-to practicalities.

In Part II of the volume, the reader explores a series of applications of social marketing to actual health behavior change projects. These projects range from ones that are national in scope to those that deal with a specific program in a given setting. The projects demonstrate that the social marketing principles are applicable to whatever level one is working at. The chapters in Part II reveal how the principles and procedures outlined in the first section are applied to the day-to-day development and administration of various health programs.

Chapter 5, by Graham Ward, details a multi-million-dollar national program designed to reduce the prevalence of uncontrolled hypertension. Ward analyzes this comprehensive project, the *National High Blood Pressure Education Program,* beginning with initial problem identification. He continues with sections on market analysis, development of the program, market segmentation, and the results and implications.

In Chapter 6, Douglas Solomon describes the community health promotion segment of the *Stanford Heart Disease Prevention Program.* Although many of the readers may be familiar with this program from its research aspects, this essay examines the project from the social marketing perspective. Solomon details the problem of heart disease and outlines two of the most significant studies performed within this project. These studies are directed toward impacting health behavior on a community-wide basis, and they illustrate the integral role of social marketing in such an effort.

The organization is the locus of intervention in Chapter 7. This chapter is coauthored by Curtis Wilbur and David Garner, and it outlines the Johnson & Johnson *Live for Life* program. This comprehensive health promotion program conducted within an organizational setting was designed to impact on employee health. The chapter highlights the considerations that went into designing this state-of-the-art program and even previews some of the early results.

Chapter 8 describes two examples of the use of marketing principles to improve the impact of health behavior change programs conducted within a single hospital setting. This chapter, coauthored by John Martin and Donald Prue, is rich with data evaluating the efforts of their approaches to improve the attendance and impact of a behavioral medicine program in a general hospital.

The chapters in Part II provide concrete examples of how social marketing principles can be applied to specific health problem areas. They also show that the application of these principles can result in programs that are both innovative and that are likely to be effective. They are programs that people will use.

The development of this volume represents the cooperation and creative efforts of many people. We gratefully acknowledge the support of our publisher and sponsoring institutions. Special thanks go to Bridget Simmerman for her unending patience in manuscript preparation. As we reflect on the individuals who have contributed most to the development of our ideas, we realize that the authors of the chapters of this book are the people who have influenced our thinking most. They have been the prime movers in making this field come alive for us. It is to the authors, for their creative efforts and persistence, that our greatest expression of appreciation must go.

LEE W. FREDERIKSEN
LAURA J. SOLOMON
KATHLEEN A. BREHONY

Contents

PART I: PRINCIPLES AND TECHNIQUES

PART II: APPLICATIONS

I
Principles and Techniques

1

Marketing Principles and Behavioral Medicine

An Overview

KATHLEEN A. BREHONY, LEE W. FREDERIKSEN, and LAURA J. SOLOMON

The dramatic increase in the human life span in the twentieth century has been largely attributed to major advancements in disease control. For example, in the United States an average of 21,000 cases of poliomyelitis per year was reported in the 5-year period before the introduction of the polio vaccine in 1955. As a result of mass immunization campaigns, the incidence of this disease was reduced to seven reported cases annually by 1974 (Berkow, 1977). Currently, there are no epidemics of polio, smallpox, cholera, leprosy, or malaria in this country, but other major health problems continue unabated.

It has become clear that most of the major remaining health problems are behaviorally based. That is, they are a result of what people do and do not do. This awareness of the relationship between behavior and health, however, is not a new idea.

Elizabeth Blackwell, the first female physician in the United States, was concerned that her contemporaries, although making contributions to society and culture, were ruining their health by their habits and life-styles. She wrote:

KATHLEEN A. BREHONY • Phobia Clinic of Southwest Virginia, Roanoke, Virginia 24016. LEE W. FREDERIKSEN • Department of Psychology, Virginia Polytechnic Institute and State University, Blacksburg, Virginia 24061. LAURA J. SOLOMON • Department of Psychology, University of Vermont, Burlington, Vermont 05405.

> Every advance in social progress removes us more and more from the guidance of instinct, obliging us to depend upon reason for the assurance that our habits are really agreeable to the laws of health, and compelling us to guard against the sacrifice of our physical or moral nature while pursuing the ends of civilization. (cited in Partnow, 1978, p. 45)

Dr. Blackwell wrote those words in 1860, but her concept is equally relevant to contemporary culture.

The belief in a strong relationship between habit and behavior on the one hand and health and sickness on the other has inspired the work of physicians, psychologists, writers, and philosophers. In fact, one of the earliest Hippocratic treatises, written *circa* 375–351 B.C., suggests the influence of daily life experiences on subsequent health or illness. Hippocrates cautioned his colleagues to consider behavioral influences in both diagnosis and treatment.

> Wherefore it appears necessary to every physician to be skilled in natures, and strive to know, if he would wish to perform his duties, what Man is in relation to the articles of food and drink, and to his other occupations, and what are the effects of each of them to every one. (cited in Hutchins, 1952, p. 7)

Epidemiological data regarding the relationship between behavior, health, and disease has advanced considerably since the writings of Hippocrates and Elizabeth Blackwell. Current information suggests that a relatively few life-style-based risk factors are potentially responsible for most of the leading causes of disease and early death. The surgeon general's 1979 report concluded as follows:

> Of the 10 leading causes of death in the United States, at least seven could be substantially reduced if persons at risk improved just five habits: diet, smoking, lack of exercise, alcohol abuse and the use of antihypertensive medication. (U.S. Department of Health, Education, and Welfare [USDHEW], 1979, p. 14)

The same surgeon general's report discusses the aggregate number of life years lost because of premature death due to chronic disease associated with social factors. These data reveal that 4.3 million years are lost due to heart disease, 833,944 years are lost due to stroke, 814,157 years are lost due to suicide, and 478,473 years are lost due to cirrhosis of the liver. In addition to the huge cost in terms of human loss, the unhealthy life-styles of the American public can be calculated in fiscal terms. In 1979, the public expenditures for health care consumed eleven cents of every federal tax dollar. The latest study by the Department of Health and Human Services projected that, even without national health insurance legislation and without adjusting for inflation, federal and private spending for health care costs increased by $78.3 billion between 1975 and 1979. That amount of spending consumed 9.1% of the gross national product (GNP), compared to 8.6% in 1975 ("Health Costs," 1979). Data compiled by the U.S. Chamber of Commerce in 1977 revealed that the average annual expenditure for health insurance paid by the companies responding to their survey was $625 per employee. This figure means that health insurance costs comprised 83% of all corporate insurance costs. Health care costs are rising at a 15%

annual rate. Costs for health care in 1983 approached $300 billion yearly—almost twice that of defense spending. These costs are expected to exceed $450 billion by 1985 and $2.4 trillion by the year 2000. Federal spending for health care costs will increase $450 billion by 1985. That amount of spending will consume over 10% of the GNP (Williams, 1983).

The data clearly indicate the tremendous human and financial costs associated with poor health. These costs must be considered in concert with other data suggesting that much of the lack of good health can be prevented by behavioral and life-style changes. Large-scale systematic efforts to alter harmful life-styles are needed if we are to become a nation of healthly people—a nation that can ultimately afford to allocate precious national resources to other areas of social development besides health care.

BEHAVIORAL MEDICINE

The notion of wholistic health, the exquisite integration of behavior and health, has been reflected in the newly found alliances between medicine and the behavioral sciences. Within the fields of psychology, medicine, and public health, the interest in health-related phenomena and the belief that the way in which people behave affects their bodies have been coalesced into a rapidly evolving subdiscipline that has been called *behavioral medicine.*

The field of behavioral medicine is still in embryonic form; thus, consensus on its definition is still forthcoming. Although a variety of definitions have been presented, the most widely accepted conceptualization of behavioral medicine was suggested by the *Yale Conference on Behavioral Medicine* (USDHEW, 1977). The conference report proposed the following definition:

> Behavioral medicine is the field concerned with the development of behavioral-science knowledge and techniques relevant to the understanding of physical health and illness and the application of this knowledge and those techniques to prevention, diagnosis, treatment and rehabilitation. Psychosis, neurosis, and substance abuse are included insofar as they contribute to physical disorders as an end point. (p. 4)

This definition is clearly a broad one, encompassing many potential activities. The actual development of the field, however, has tended to follow four general lines of approach (Pomerleau & Brady, 1979). The first of these involves therapeutic interventions aimed at directly changing a problem behavior or symptom. Examples of such interventions include the use of electromyography (EMG) biofeedback to reduce muscle tension associated with tension headaches. EMG biofeedback may also be useful in muscular reeducation with individuals who have lost muscular control following a stroke. The systematic use of rewards and punishment (contingency management) has also found application in the modification of problematic behaviors such as vomiting by individuals with anorexia nervosa and increasing activity levels in individuals with chronic pain. In all of the preceding examples, behavioral procedures are applied to the modification of a problem behavior or symptom in an individual patient.

A second line of development in behavioral medicine focuses on interventions directed toward the behavior of health care providers rather than patients directly. The assumption is that by changing the behavior of the health care provider, one can have a much broader impact than by focusing only on individual patients. Examples of such interventions include the development of materials to assist physicians in helping their hypertensive patients stop smoking, the training of health care personnel to conduct more effective interviews, and the establishment of efficient patient tracking procedures to monitor patients' progress and to provide feedback to the health professional. The *National High Blood Pressure Education Program,* described elsewhere in this volume, is an excellent example of the application of this general approach (Solomon, 1982).

A third line of development focuses on the use of behavioral techniques to improve patient compliance with other forms of medical treatment. Examples of this include the application of contingent reinforcers to ensure that patients take medication in prescribed amounts at the right times, the use of telephone or written prompts to increase appointment keeping at dental visits, and the introduction of self-monitoring to facilitate adherence to a therapeutic diet or exercise regimen. The *National High Blood Pressure Education Program* provides a good example of how these strategies have been used.

The fourth line of development is aimed at disease prevention and health promotion. Common examples of this approach involve the modification of risk factors for a variety of disorders. The elimination of cigarette smoking, the reduction in serum cholesterol levels, the increase in exercise, the reduction of sodium intake, and the management of stress are all examples of a preventive approach. The goal here is to prevent disease by the reduction of targeted risk factors. During recent years there has also been an increased emphasis on the promotion of positive health rather than simply the prevention of disease. *Health promotion* refers to the development of behaviors that improve bodily functioning and enhance an individual's ability to adapt to a changing environment. In other words, health is not simply the absence of disease. Rather, it is a positive state that the individual must actively pursue rather than passively experience. The goal of health promotion is becoming a dominant thrust in many health programs, and must clearly be considered an essential component in behavioral medicine.

It seems clear that behavioral medicine has many potential contributions to offer. However if this promise is to be fulfilled, there are at least two limits that must be overcome. First, too often programs are not designed with an eye toward their acceptance by consumers. This can result in programs that may incorporate proven, state-of-the-art techniques but that suffer from the dual problems of low acceptance by potential consumers and high dropout rates among participants. Although examples of this type of program abound, programs in the areas of weight management (Stunkard, 1979) and smoking cessation (Bernstein & Glasgow, 1979; Frederiksen & Simon, 1979) are prime examples.

A closely related but somewhat different problem involves the acceptance of programs by the intermediaries or health professionals who must actually deliver the intervention. For example, through research we may determine that an admonition to stop smoking delivered by a health professional is an effective way to motivate patients to change their smoking behavior. However, we are then faced with the task of ensuring that the health professionals actually deliver that admonition to the appropriate patients. If they do not accept the procedure of delivering this admonition, an otherwise effective approach is rendered useless.

These two factors—the failure to design programs in ways that are acceptable to consumers and the failure to stimulate relevant intermediaries to use the procedures effectively—present limitations to the ultimate effectiveness of behavioral medicine interventions. However, it is our thesis that there are approaches that can overcome these barriers.

MARKETING FOR HEALTH-RELATED BEHAVIORS

One method for reducing the culture lag or the reluctance of large numbers of people to engage in healthy life-style behaviors may lie in our abilities to market these life-style changes effectively. The successful integration of marketing strategies and behavior change strategies holds tremendous promise for the reduction of life-style-based health problems. The remainder of this chapter will address the issue of effective marketing principles and behavior change strategies, the ethics of marketing within a professional framework, the limitations of marketing strategies for health promotion, and some common misconceptions (e.g., confusion between marketing and selling or advertising).

Kotter and Zaltman (1971) articulated the notion that marketing strategies might be effectively applied to areas other than commercial products or services. These authors noted that regardless of the content area, *social marketing,* or the marketing of socially relevant programs, ideas, or behaviors, is concerned with "the design, implementation, and control of programs calculated to include the acceptability of social ideas and involving considerations of product planning, pricing, communication, distribution and marketing research" (p. 6). Thus, marketing emphasizes a voluntary exchange process that incorporates several processes, such as (1) the development of a clear-cut plan and objectives that determine specific strategies; (2) market segmentation or the determination of consumers and potential consumers; (3) key consumer benefits or a justification of why the consumer should buy the product; and (4) "product personality," or the identification of products across a variety of presentation styles.

The strategies employed by professional marketers have been successful in inducing people to behave in certain ways as consumers of various commercial products and services. These same strategies can serve to facilitate behavioral change for the purposes of health promotion and other social issues. In 1952, G. D. Wiebe asked, "Why can't you sell brotherhood like you sell soap?" (quoted in Kotler, 1975, p. 286) As Kotler and Zaltman (1971) have pointed out, this question implies that sellers of soap are generally more effective than "sellers" of social causes. Indeed, Wiebe's (1951–1952) data revealed that social (health) campaigns were successful to the extent that their techniques resembled those of a commercial product campaign. If this is indeed the case, then it would be of value to observe the marketing strategies utilized by the specialists who have been selling us toothpaste, soap powder, and cigarettes. From this information, we can learn process principles of effective large-scale behavior change. Although it is unlikely that marketing concepts can be incorporated wholesale into health promotion strategies, it is possible that appropriate translations can be undertaken. Limitations of marketing strategies for health promotion will be outlined later in this chapter. First let us look at some areas of applicability of marketing techniques. As we shall see, the use of marketing strategies for health promotion introduces some new concepts to the behavioral scientist. However, many marketing concepts and strategies are outgrowths of principles the behavioral scientist knows quite well.

Market Research

Market research incorporates five basic steps (Kotler, 1975). These steps include problem definition, research design, fieldwork, data analysis, and report preparation. The first step, *problem definition,* is a similar concept to what behavioral scientists would term *operationalizing the problem.* That is, the problem should be defined in a specific and testable manner. For example, Kotler (1975) cites the case of an administrator in the U.S. Postal Service who asked a market researcher to find out everything he or she could about attitudes toward the U.S. Postal Service. This objective would be something like asking a behavioral scientist to determine why people live unhealthy life-styles. Phrasing empirical questions in broad and amorphous ways does not allow for the development of evaluation strategies that can provide useful answers to important questions.

The second step for effective market research, according to Kotler, is the *research design* phase. This step is concerned with data collection methods, research instruments, and sampling plan. In this case, even the marketing language is identical to concepts that the behavioral scientist would consider in the empirical investigation of a research question. Market researchers are aware of primary and secondary data sources, the use of observation, experimentation, and surveys as methods to obtain these data as well as the importance of reliable and valid research instruments. Similarly, Kotler notes that *effective data analysis,* the third step in market research, attempts to extract meaningful information from the data through statistical techniques such as correlation analysis, multiple regression, discriminant analysis, factor analysis, and cluster analysis.

The concepts and even the language used to describe effective market research are identical, in most cases, to what the behavioral scientist has developed for effective assessment of the behavioral phenomena that he or she has chosen to investigate. In fact, if we were to substitute the term *needs assessment* in place of *market research,* it becomes clear that the market researcher and the behavioral scientist utilize very similar conceptualizations and methodologies. Thus, the transition to this marketing strategy for the purpose of marketing health-related behaviors does not require a conceptual shift for the behavioral scientist. What we can learn from the marketing profession, instead, are new and potentially valuable sources of primary and secondary data.

Market Segmentation

Market segmentation has been defined as "dividing the market into fairly homogeneous parts where any part may conceivably be selected as a market target to be reached with a distinct marketing mix" (Kotler, 1975, p. 99). It is clear that no product, service, or health promotion campaign can be successful if it attempts to be all things to all people. The use of market segmentation strategies is respectful of the fact that those in the market do not all have the same intensity of interest in the product nor do they have equal resources. Market segmentation may rely on demographic or behavioral differences among groups.

Commercial sector products and services appear to have carried this concept to a very sophisticated state-of-the-art level. One need only think of familiar television commercials or magazine advertisements to understand the extent to which professional marketers attempt to penetrate or reach a certain and specific subset of their potential market.

Figures 1 and 2 show two magazine advertisements for the same product—cigarettes. With the exception of the notification of the Surgeon General's Office, which is required by law, neither of these ads talks about the salient health facts regarding cigarettes as we know them (i.e., that cigarettes have been identified as a major risk factor in lung cancer and cardiovascular disease). Instead, these ads reflect the marketing observation "sell the sizzle, not the steak." And the "sizzle" for these very similar products is presented in very different ways. The Virginia Slims advertisement is directed to a particular segment of women. This cigarette is not for all women but for "liberated" women who perhaps see themselves as independent, tasteful, and successful. The product definition or identity does not stop with the advertisement itself. The packaging of the product and the actual size and shape of the cigarette (product) are "slimmer than the fat cigarettes men smoke." The Marl-

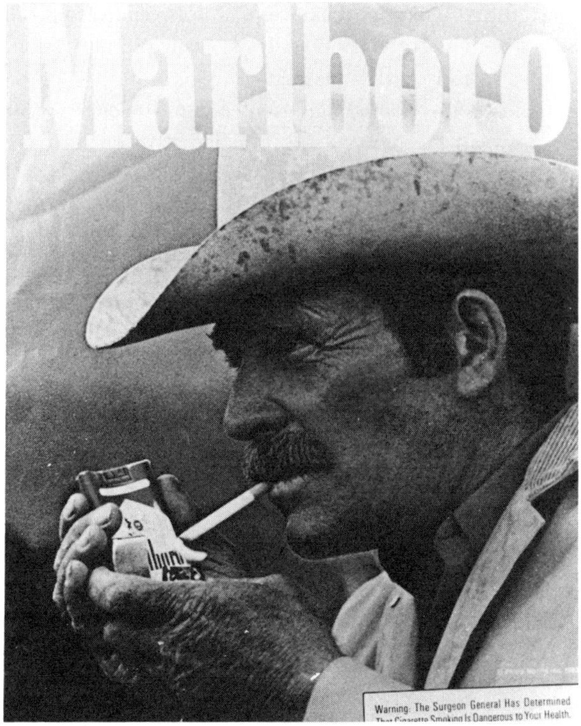

Figure 1. Marlboro advertisement. (Copyright 1983 by Philip Morris Inc., New York. Reprinted by permission.)

boro advertisement, on the other hand, shows a man who, we might assume, is not at all concerned about the size and shape of his cigarette. Instead, we see an individual who wants good taste. He is rugged, assertive, masculine, and clearly in charge. Imagine, if you will, the Marlboro man trying to promote Virginia Slims cigarettes, and you will understand how carefully and specifically Madison Avenue defines market segments.

Figure 3 shows a can of Campbell's soup, a product that has been familiar to most of us for many years. You will notice that this soup can is a little different from the one that you saw as a child. The familiar red and white label is still there, but a tag has been added. The tag identifies this soup as "one of the light ones." However, this is not a new product; this soup is one of the old standbys. Although the soup has not changed, the targeted audience has. Campbell recently labeled all its products having fewer than 100 calories as "one of the light ones" in order to appeal to a newly emerging market segment—individuals concerned about weight control. One might assume that this product is competing for the market segment that would also purchase other low-calorie products. If the large-scale interest in light eating con-

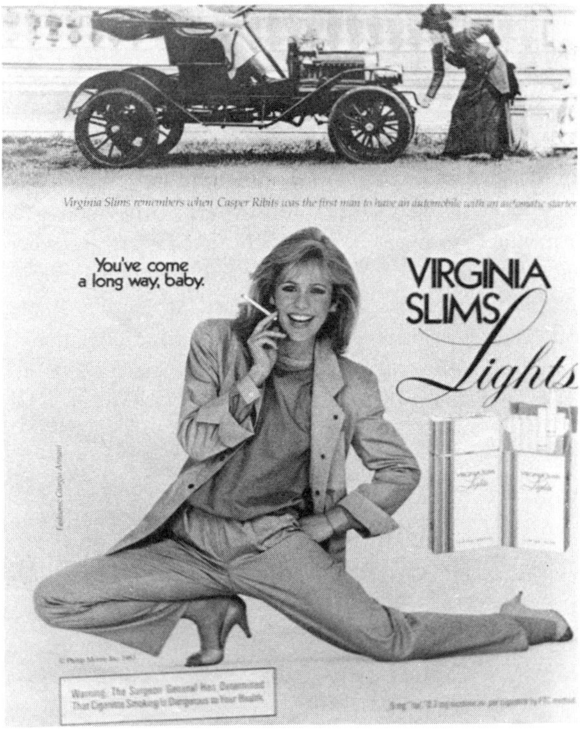

Figure 2. Virginia Slims advertisement. (Copyright 1983 by Philip Morris Inc., New York. Reprinted by permission.)

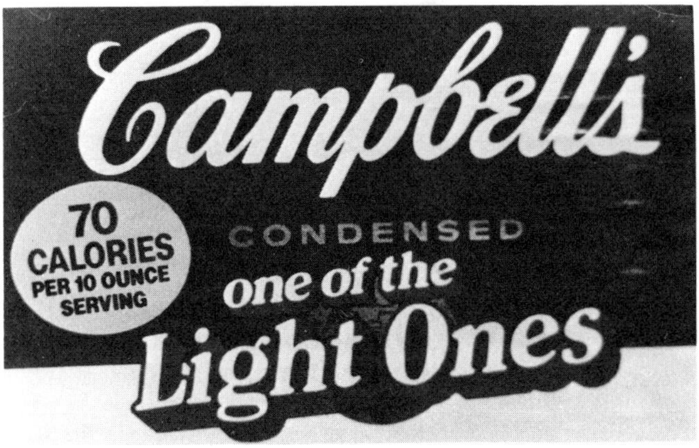

Figure 3. Campbell's soup label. (Reprinted by permission of Campbell Soup Company, Camden, New Jersey.)

tinues, we are likely to see such commercial products as low-calorie fast-food soybean burgers or "Tofu Helper"!

The notion of market segmentation has been developed to sophisticated levels by marketing experts. However, the concept should be familiar to behavioral scientists who have called their version of this construct *target populations*. The specifics of any particular health behavior change program, like other more tangible products, are not likely to appeal to everyone. Unfortunately, behavioral scientists have not fine tuned their products to match the needs of specific target audiences with quite the same precision as our marketing counterparts. A noteworthy exception is the emphasis on high blood pressure control with black Americans. In order to reach and impact this large market segment, many of the educational materials are clearly directed toward a black audience. Figure 4 shows a poster that depicts this strategy of targeting blacks as a distinctive market segment for the product (e.g., information).

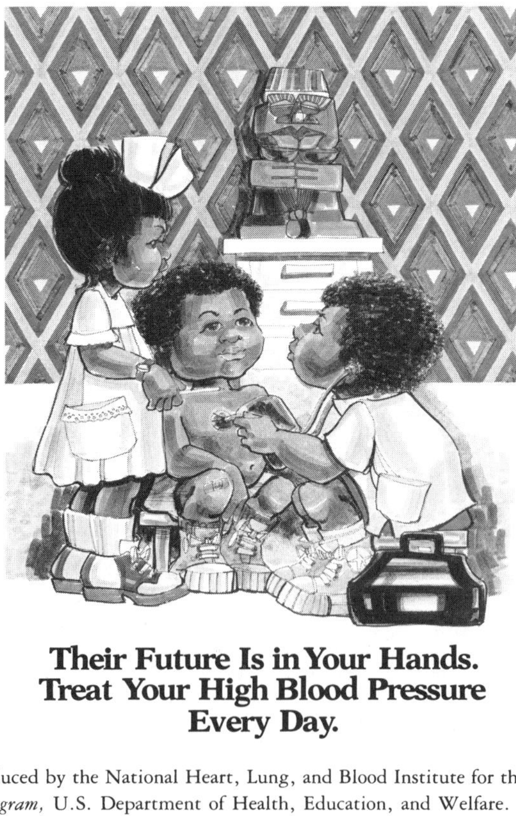
Their Future Is in Your Hands.
Treat Your High Blood Pressure
Every Day.

Figure 4. Poster produced by the National Heart, Lung, and Blood Institute for the *National High Blood Pressure Education Program,* U.S. Department of Health, Education, and Welfare.

Consumer Benefit

Marketing specialists design campaigns around the rule of thumb that every successful campaign must understand and meet the needs of the consumer. Kotler (1975) pointed out the following:

> Marketing relies on designing the organization's offering in terms of the target market's needs and desires rather than in terms of the seller's personal tastes. Marketing is a democratic rather than elitist technology. It holds that efforts are likely to fail that try to impose on a market a product, service or idea that is not matched to the market's tastes or desires. (pp. 6–7)

The four key psychological variables that appear to make up complex consumer behavior are (1) the need of the market, (2) the perception of the market with regard to the offering as well as the organization, (3) the preferences of consumers among a set of alternative offerings, and (4) the satisfaction of the consumer with the offering. All of these variables present both the professional marketer and the behavioral scientist with empirical issues that must be assessed.

Behavioral scientists will notice the similarity between the notions of *consumer benefit* and *reinforcement.* That is, what does the consumer (or patient, client, community group, weight reduction class, and so forth) perceive as the reward for engaging in the designated behavior? The reinforcing properties of any program must be considered against the response costs to the individual for participating in the consumption of that product or service. Response cost may be defined as the removal of previously acquired reinforcers contingent upon a response (Craighead, Kazdin, & Mahoney, 1976). For example, participants in stress management workshops are generally asked to absorb several costs, including (1) a monetary fee for participating, (2) the time needed to attend the workshops that had been devoted to other activities, and (3) the transportation hassles that arise from needing to get to the right place at the right time. The professional marketing expert as well as the behavioral scientist must find ways of identifying (or creating) salient reinforcers to offset these response costs.

Although there are many similarities between effective marketing in the commercial sector and the marketing of health-related social programs, there are some important differences. Purchasing a commercial sector product generally requires less time and effort than is required when making a major life-style and health behavior change. For example, many consumer products rely on an individual's being aware of the benefits of a product at the point-of-purchase stage. That is, an individual shops for toothpaste and makes a decision to purchase Crest or Gleem. The marketing strategy behind the purchase of toothpaste has not been to convince the public that brushing one's teeth is a good behavior. Instead, the behavior of brushing one's teeth on a daily basis is defined and supported by cultural norms of hygiene, cleanliness, and attractiveness. The toothpaste marketer has only to convince the individual that one particular product will have better results than another.

The behavioral scientist wishing to change life-style behaviors is up against a very different set of circumstances. For example, a professional attempting to reduce sodium intake among hypertensives in a community setting must compete against all the good-tasting and popular foods with high-sodium content. Individuals who are interested in seriously reducing their sodium intake must make substantial modifications in everyday behavior, and they must do this consistently. The response cost in this example is quite high. First of all, the individual must become a label reader in order to learn which foods contain large and small amounts of sodium. Many of this culture's most popular prepared foods are very high in sodium content, and alternative foods may not be as palatable or as comparable in price as their high-sodium counterparts. This individual would be confronted with a difficult problem when eating out, because most restaurants do not identify low- or high-sodium foods. The response cost in complying with a low-sodium diet is considerably higher than the more specific behavior of purchasing a particular brand of toothpaste. Additionally, the positive effects of maintaining a low-sodium diet are not immediately apparent. Hypertension is an asymptomatic disease, and there is not an immediate or discernible improvement in how one feels as a result of maintaining the new behavior pattern (e.g., sodium restriction). Thus, in this example, short-term benefits of life-style change are not particularly rewarding and the long-term benefits (of improved health) may not appear to be "worth all the trouble."

The behavioral scientist interested in using marketing strategies for health promotion must be acutely aware of the importance of programming in as many short-term consumer benefits (reinforcers) as possible. Although this may seem like a Herculean task, it is also an opportunity for creative application of what we know about the principles of behavior. For example, a growing number of restaurants, in conjunction with the American Heart Association, are identifying low-calorie, low-sodium, and low-cholesterol menu entrées by placing a small picture of a heart next to those items on the menu. One can imagine that this intervention is making it easier to select healthy foods by providing attractive alternatives and by telling the consumer which meals are prepared according to what dietary considerations. The cost to the restaurant may be relatively low because the cost of printing a small logo next to certain items will not substantially increase the price of menu printing. In fact, the restaurant is likely to be viewed in a very positive way by individuals who are interested in complying with certain dietary restrictions.

Another example highlighting immediate consumer benefit while reducing response costs is to modify the place in which consumers purchase the service or product. Adelphi University provided the commuters on the Long Island Railroad with an opportunity to participate in a stress management program while they were traveling home after work. This is an excellent example of enhancing consumer benefit, especially when the alternative method of delivery is considered. A busy worker in New York who wanted to take a training course in stress management delivered in a more traditional mode would be likely to rush home from work, choke down dinner, arrange for a baby-sitter, get in the car, and drive to a community mental health center or other location to learn to relax and cope with stress more effectively. It is not difficult to see that, in this example, participation in the stress management program is likely to make this individual even more stressed, at least on the days that the training was held! An individual required to engage in this chain of behaviors is likely to lose interest and become noncompliant—a major problem with most health behavior interventions. The recognition of the needs of the consumer created an impetus to design a creative and nontraditional delivery system for this particular stress management program.

Specialists in marketing believe that, just as successful campaigns demonstrate a salient consumer benefit, successful campaigns rarely scold or threaten but usually promise a reward that people want and need (Martin, 1979). Thus, effective health promotion campaigns, in general, should highlight the positive consequences of disease-reducing behaviors. Although this direction is consistent with the basic principles of marketing, it continues to be open to study with regard to the marketing of health promotion programs.

PRODUCT PERSONALITY AND THE OTHER THREE *P*'S

Professional marketers like to speak of the four basic concerns for any product or service campaign as the four *p*'s: product, price, promotion, and place. These basic marketing concepts define what will be termed the *marketing mix.* We will discuss each of these in turn with an eye toward their applicability to the behavioral scientist interested in the promotion of health.

Product

The term *product* is used to define physical objects, services, persons, places, organizations, and ideas. It is critical that the product be described in very concrete and specific terms because this affects the size and composition of the market. As Kotler (1975) points out:

> If the product is defined as health service, then the market consists of everyone in the world. If the product is defined as a smokers' clinic, then the market consists of everyone who smokes. If the product is defined as a smokers' clinic that meets weekly Tuesday evenings at the Passavant Hospital in Chicago, then the market consists of all smokers who might find this product assessible. If the product is defined as the same clinic charging $1,000 for treatment, then the market consists of all smokers who find this product assessible and the price acceptable. The more specifically the product is defined, the smaller is the market size. Also, the less attractively the product is defined, the smaller is the market size. (p. 95)

Solomon (1979) observed that a product or service can be defined as the "focus of the transaction which takes place in marketing between the marketer and the target audience" (p. 10). Products of interest to behavioral scientists are frequently more complex and difficult to define than products marketed by the commercial sector. For example, the core generic product of the *Stanford Heart Disease Prevention Program* as well as the *National High Blood Pressure Education Program* is information. Some of this product (i.e., information) is intangible and is offered through various media channels such as television and radio. Other information comes in more tangible form, such as booklets and audiocassettes. Solomon (1979), in describing the product line of the Stanford program, noted that "formative research and planning processes contribute to the careful conceptualization and design of all of these products" (p. 10). The objective of the Stanford program is to change behaviors that have been identified as risk factors in cardiovascular disease. In defining and developing the product line, attention was focused on the original goals of the program. Several considerations formed the basis for all product development. First, decisions were made regarding which aspects of heart disease prevention and which benefits of preventive actions would be emphasized in all of the materials. Secondly, consideration was given to the positioning of the product with regard to competing behaviors that people might engage in as well as with regard to competing products (e.g., commercially available smoking cessation programs, Weight Watchers). Thirdly, decisions were made about which combinations of coronary risk factors would be the focus of materials and programs (e.g., smoking, weight reduction, nutritional concerns). Finally, the product line was oriented not only toward the key target group (individuals at risk for coronary heart disease) but also to secondary groups such as health professionals, community organizations, and retailers (Solomon, 1979).

Kotler (1975) noted five major dimensions that should be considered in the conceptualization of any product. These dimensions include durability (how long the product lasts), complexity (how complicated the product is), and visibility (how conspicuous the product is). For example, the behavioral scientist interested in weight reduction as a method of reducing health risk has a variety of products from which to choose. Two very different products might be (1) a behavior change program that attempts to break unhealthy eating patterns by encouraging consumption of low-calorie foods in certain places or at specific times, stimulus control over types of food allowed in the house, alteration of actual eating behaviors such as chewing food more slowly and putting utensils down between bites, and increased exercise; or (2) intestinal bypass surgery.

With regard to the various product dimensions of durability, complexity, visibility, risk, and familiarity, we can imagine that these two products would differ quite a bit. The behavior change strategy is less durable compared to the surgical intervention. The behavior change strategy is less complex and less risky, although it is also more visible and more familiar. These two products, like all products, are described in comparative terms. In defining and developing new products, it is necessary to determine the attributes that the identified market segment would ideally like to see. In this particular case, it is likely that intestinal bypass surgery would suggest too great a response cost, too high a risk, and would be too unfamiliar a procedure to be marketed successfully to a wide target market (e.g., individuals at risk for health problems because of their obesity). There is, however, likely to be some market segment for whom the surgical intervention might be appropriate and acceptable. Thus, the product changes, depending on the target audience.

Price

In his discussion regarding price considerations, Kotler (1975) quotes Adam Smith as saying: "The real price of everything, what everything really costs to the man who wants to acquire it, is the toil and trouble of acquiring it" (p. 176). Price considerations are particularly relevant in the health promotion field because many of the costs are not financial. Price, in this regard, can be equated with the behavioral notion of response cose, and it includes monetary costs as well as psychological costs, social costs, and costs in terms of time and effort. Additionally, health promoters working in the public sector (e.g., government) have very different mandates than those working in the private sector. For example, private sector companies can easily ignore marketing to less-profitable market segments, whereas public sector programs are often specifically designed to target these hard-to-reach segments.

Place

Another component of the marketing mix is place of distribution. This concerns how the organization plans to make its products and services available and accessible to consumers. The previously cited example of delivery of stress management programs to commuters on the Long Island Railroad is an excellent example of creative distribution decisions.

Consider some additional examples. The *Stanford Heart Disease Prevention Program* used diversified distribution channels in order to reach a broadly defined market (i.e., all those at risk for cardiovascular disease in certain communities). The Stanford distribution channels included mass media, health professionals, community organizations, and commercial networks. The concern was to provide the target market with multiple opportunities, places, and forums for obtaining information and for achieving self-directed behavior change. However even within this broad-based effort, the market segmentation helped to determine how the product would be defined and how it would be distributed. Information regarding smoking as a risk factor for health was presented in a very different way when it was aimed at teenagers and discussed in a public service announcement (PSA) on a top-40 radio station than when it was directed toward business executives in an organizational setting.

Here are some examples of distribution. Brehony, Geller, Benson, and Solomon (1980) designed a procedure to recruit volunteer subjects for a research and treatment study on agoraphobia. Market research (e.g., review of the empirical literature) revealed the promotional channels that would be most cost-effective in recruiting subjects. The literature indicated that the majority of agoraphobic individuals are middle-aged, middle-class women who are not employed outside their homes. With limited time and resources with which to promote this treatment and research project, decisions were made to reach the target population by way of television talk shows that were aired during the day and newspaper articles placed on the feature and women's pages. This strategy proved very effective in reaching the target audience.

The majority of cases of venereal disease are among homosexual males. This is attributed to cultural and life-style behaviors among this particular target population. An innovative distribution strategy involved the availability of blood tests and other assessment procedures at gay bars. This project arranged with owners of the bars to allow a physician and laboratory technician to set up a lab in a private space. The venereal disease screening was available to anyone interested in participating.

In organizational settings (e.g., Johnson & Johnson), employees are offered health promotion education on company time. During work breaks, employees may participate in I-quit-smoking classes instead of consuming their usual coffee and cigarettes.

Alcoholism treatment programs (e.g., Compcare) offer alcohol-free parties on New Year's Eve for recovering alcoholics. The place of distribution, in this example, may be thought of as a time of distribution, because New Year's Eve is closely associated with alcohol in our culture. Thus, it is a major risk period for becoming noncompliant with abstinence or controlled-drinking goals.

All of the distribution decisions must be made with an eye toward the needs of the market, definition of the product, and cost considerations. The Stanford program and the *National High Blood Pressure Education Program* cannot, for example, hire a group of technicians to be available on-call to deliver information about risk reduction to individuals or individual families interested in learning about health promotion. As Kotler (1975) has pointed out, the product is typically removed in space from the location of the consumer and in time according to when the consumer would like to use it. Thus, creative strategies for distribution of the product must be incorporated into health promotion campaigns.

Promotion

"Promotion is a form of communication that encompasses all the tools of the marketing mix whose major role is persuasive communication" (Kotler, 1975 p. 201). Promotional tools include advertising, publicity, personal contact, incentives, and atmospherics (efforts to design the place of purchase to create specific cognitive or emotional effects in consumers). People frequently confuse promotion—one component of the entire marketing strategy—with marketing itself. In many minds, marketing and advertising are one and the same. In fact, advertising is only one aspect of marketing and only one of several forms of promotion.

The differences between commercial sector marketing and health promotion marketing become very clear when we consider promotion of a product or service. For example, behavioral scientists are bound by rules of professional ethics to promote their programs in clearly defined ways. Frequently, there are little or no resources for promotion. For example, advertising (one element of promotion) in the commerical world is a mainstay of marketing programs, and although it is coming into greater use in the nonprofit sector, this is a relatively new phenomenon.

Decisions regarding product, price, place, and promotion are not mutually exclusive events. Instead, these concerns must be considered simultaneously. Product definition will, in some respects, be determined by price considerations, by where the product can be delivered, and by opportunities for promotion. The behavioral scientist interested in health promotion, like the marketer of commercial products, must consider each of these variables and simultaneously adjust marketing strategies. As Kotler (1975) points out, each *p* is in reality a collection of instruments, and each is sufficiently complex to warrant a lifetime of specialization. Thus, there are specialists in product design, in pricing, in distribution, and in promotion. The general marketer knows the basics of all these instruments and blends them in preparing a marketing plan. Like the more general marketer, the behavioral scientist must become something of a generalist and understand at least the basics of these important marketing principles in order to impact effectively on health-related behaviors.

The discussion of the basic principles of marketing has, we hope, illustrated some of the similarities and differences between the field of marketing and the behavioral sciences. Some of this information appears to be new to the behavioral scientist. However, many of the major marketing basics are conceptually compatible with what behavioral scientists already know. For example, the notion of consumer benefit is similar to reinforcement and response cost considerations. Market segmentation parallels the notion of target populations. In some ways, the behavioral scientist who is interested in the use of marketing strategies must learn a new literature and a new way of conceptualizing issues. In other ways, he or she must simply learn a new system of technical language rather than make a major paradigm shift.

It is unlikely that behavioral scientists will begin to sell health promotion in the way that kitchen gadgets are sold on late-night television. There are some fundamental differences between what is possible in marketing commercial sector products and marketing health behavior change. Restrictions come from ethical concerns as well as the different needs and mandates of commercial and nonprofit organizations.

Bloom and Novelli (1981) have addressed some of the very real problems in applying traditional marketing strategies to social causes. These writers have noted:

> While the authors believe strongly in the contribution marketing can make to social programs, they feel compelled to temper the enthusiasm that they may have shown for social marketing by pointing out the difficulties and challenges associated with its practice. (p. 79)

Readers are referred to this excellent article for a detailed discussion of these issues. In brief, the authors discuss comparisons between commercial marketing and social marketing with regard to the following aspects:

1. Market analysis
   (a) Social marketers generally have less good secondary data available about their consumers.
   (b) Social marketers have more difficulty obtaining valid, reliable measures of salient variables.
   (c) Social marketers have more difficulty sorting out the relative influence of identified determinants of consumer behavior.
   (d) Social marketers have more difficulty getting consumer research studies funded, approved, and completed in a timely fashion.
2. Market segmentation problems
   (a) Social marketers face pressure against segmentation, in general, and especially against segmentation that leads to ignoring of certain segments.
   (b) Social marketers frequently do not have accurate behavioral data to use in identifying segments.
   (c) Social marketers' target segments must often consist of those consumers who are the most negatively predisposed to their offerings.
3. Product strategy problems
   (a) Social marketers tend to have less flexibility in shaping their products or offerings.
   (b) Social marketers have more difficulty in formulating product concepts.
   (c) Social marketers have more difficulty selecting and implementing long-term positioning strategies.
4. Pricing strategy problems
   (a) Social marketers find that the development of a pricing strategy primarily involves trying to reduce the monetary, psychic, energy, and time costs incurred by consumers when engaging in a desired social behavior.
   (b) Social marketers have difficulties measuring their prices because they tend to have less control over consumer costs.
5. Channels (intermediaries) strategy problems
   (a) Social marketers have more difficulty utilizing and controlling desired intermediaries.

6. Communications strategy problems
   (a) Social marketers usually find paid advertising impossible to use.
   (b) Social marketers usually must communicate relatively large amounts of information in their messages.
   (c) Social marketers have difficulty conducting meaningful pretests of messages.
7. Organizational design and planning problems
   (a) Social marketers must function in organizations where marketing activities are poorly understood, weakly appreciated, and inappropriately located.
   (b) Social marketers must function in organizations where plans (if any are developed) are treated as archival rather than action documents.
   (c) Social marketers must predict how both friendly and unfriendly competitors will behave.
8. Evaluation problems
   (a) Social marketers frequently face difficulties trying to define effectiveness measures.
   (b) Social marketers often find it difficult to estimate the contribution their marketing program has made toward the achievement of certain objectives.

Bloom and Novelli (1981) conclude by noting the following:

> We have attempted to document why social marketing (compared to commercial marketing) is the more difficult game to master. While success in the battles over market share in industries like detergents or automobiles may call for equal or even greater stamina and perserverance, success in the social marketing arena requires greater ingenuity and imagination. (p. 87)

This chapter has attempted to point out the possibilities for social marketing strategies in their application to large-scale health promotion efforts. However, it does appear that marketing concepts cannot be adopted wholesale by health promotion programs. Solomon (1979, p. 2) noted that "Wiebe was wrong. You *cannot* sell brotherhood like you sell soap." Although this is true, it is also possible that by recognizing the marketing principles that *can* be used in better accomplishing health behavior change we can take the strategies that once urged the consumer to "walk a mile for a Camel" and now urge consumers to just "walk a mile."

SUMMARY

This chapter began with the recognition that many medical disorders leading to premature death and disability can be linked in part to life-style behaviors. We then discussed the emergence of behavioral medicine, a new discipline composed of professionals from the behavioral sciences and medical communities. Despite advances in the field, we are not yet particularly effective in promoting widespread changes in health-related behavior. One promising approach to this dilemma is the systematic application of marketing principles to the task of changing health-related behaviors. The area of social marketing is the conceptual base for this effort. Some of the major principles of a marketing approach were reviewed, and special attention was given to how these principles are similar to concepts already known in the behavioral sciences. Finally, some of the limitations of the social marketing approach were briefly discussed.

REFERENCES

Berkow, R. (Ed.). *The Merck manual.* Rahway, N.J.: Sharpe and Dohme Research Laboratories, 1977.

Bernstein, D. A., & Glasgow, R. E. Smoking. In O. F. Pomerleau & J. P. Brady (Eds.), *Behavioral medicine: Theory and practice.* Baltimore: Williams & Wilkins, 1979.

Bloom, P. N., & Novelli, W. D. Problems and challenges of social marketing. *Journal of Marketing,* 1981, *45,* 79–88.

Brehony, K. A., Geller, E. S., Benson, B. A., & Solomon, L. J. *Epidemiological data and agoraphobia: An American sample.* Unpublished manuscript, Virginia Polytechnic Institute and State University, 1980.

Craighead, W. E., Kazdin, A. E., & Mahoney, M. J. *Behavior modification: Principles, issues and applications.* Boston: Houghton Mifflin Co., 1976.

Frederiksen, L. W., & Simon, S. J. Modification of smoking behavior. In R. S. Davidson (Ed.), *Modification of pathological behavior.* New York: Gardner Press, 1979.

Health costs: What limit? *Time,* May 28, 1979, pp. 60–68.

Hutchins, R. M. *Great books of the western world: Vol. 10. Hippocrates and Galen.* Chicago: Encyclopaedia Britannica, Inc., 1952.

Kotler, P. *Marketing for non-profit organizations.* Englewood Cliffs, N.J.: Prentice-Hall, 1975.

Kotler, P., & Zaltman, G. Social marketing: An approach to planned social change. *Journal of Marketing,* July 1971, pp. 3–12.

Martin, G. Personal communication, September 1979.

Partnow, E. *The quotable woman.* Garden City, N.Y.: Anchor Press, 1978.

Pomerleau, O. F., & Brady, J. P. *Behavioral medicine: Theory and practice.* Baltimore: Williams & Wilkins, 1979.

Solomon, D. S. *Social marketing and health promotion: The Stanford Heart Disease Prevention Program community studies.* Paper presented to the Association for the Advancement of Behavior Therapy, San Francisco, December 1979.

Solomon, L. J. Personal communication, August 5, 1982.

Stunkard, A. J. Behavioral medicine and beyond: The example of obesity. In O. F. Pomerleau & J. P. Brady (Eds.), *Behavioral medicine: Theory and practice.* Baltimore: Williams & Wilkins, 1979.

U.S. Department of Health, Education, and Welfare. *Healthy people: The surgeon general's report on health promotion and disease prevention.* Washington, D.C.: U.S. Government Printing Office, 1979.

U.S. Department of Health, Education and Welfare. *Yale conference on behavioral medicine.* Washington, D.C.: U.S. Government Printing Office, 1977.

Wiebe, G. D. Merchandising commodities and citizenship on television. *Public Opinion Quarterly,* Winter 1951–1952, pp. 679–691.

Williams, L. W. Rx needed: First aid for rising health care costs. *P.P.G. Products Magazine,* 1983, *91,* 1.

2

Social Marketing of Health Behavior

PHILIP KOTLER

We are coming to recognize that there is a marketplace of ideas just as there is a marketplace of goods. Examples abound of organizations striving to motivate the public to adopt a new idea or practice. For example, the National Safety Council wants people to wear their safety belts when driving, and the American Cancer Society wants people to stop smoking. The American Medical Association wants people to take an annual physical checkup, the New York Police Department wants people to lock their car doors, and the National Organization for Women wants men to view women as equals.

These efforts to alter the beliefs, attitudes, values, or behavior of target groups have different names. They are called *propaganda* efforts by their critics and *educational* efforts by their supporters. They are perfectly normal activities and are found in all societies. Every group has its cause and actively attempts to market its viewpoint to others. In a totalitarian society, only one group is allowed to propagate openly for official causes. In a free society, all groups propagate their viewpoints in the marketplace of ideas.

Idea marketers are known by many names—propagandists, agitators, charismatic leaders, publicists, lobbyists, change agents, and so on. Many of them see their task in narrow terms, as that of developing and disseminating persuasive messages. We shall argue, however, that effective communication is only one part of the total task required to market an idea successfully. The adoption of an idea, like

Philip Kotler, *Marketing for Nonprofit Organizations,* 2nd ed., © 1982. Adapted by permission of Prentice-Hall, Inc., Englewood Cliffs, N.J.

PHILIP KOTLER • J. L. Kellogg Graduate School of Management, Northwestern University, Evanston, Illinois 60201.

the adoption of any product, requires a deep understanding of the needs, perceptions, preferences, reference groups, and behavioral patterns of the target audience, and it requires the tailoring of messages, media, costs, and facilities to maximize the ease of adopting the idea. We use the term *social marketing* for these tasks. We believe that social marketing provides an effective conceptual system for thinking through the problems of bringing about changes in the ideas or practices of a target public.

Before proceeding however, it is desirable to answer the objection that social marketing provides Machiavellian guidance on how to get people to do what they do not want to do; that is, it provides a means of social manipulation and control. In the first place, it is a very difficult task to change people for good or bad. Those who work in face-to-face relations with individual clients and have their trust, such as psychologists, physicians, social workers, or relatives, know how difficult it is to change another person. It is even more difficult to change a whole group of people when the means are mass media that appear infrequently. Although social marketing attempts to harness the insights of behavioral science and exchange theory to the task of social change, its power to bring about actual change, or to bring it about in a reasonable amount of time, is highly limited. The greater the target group's investment in a value or behavioral pattern, the more resistant it is to change. Social marketing works best in situations where the type of change counts the least.

Second, social marketing takes place in society whether or not its methods are openly described. Some groups will be better at it than others. Rather than keep social marketing methodology a deep secret and thus leave certain groups at a disadvantage, this methodology should be openly discussed and examined. This will allow both sides of an issue to formulate improved plans as well as alert the public to how groups market a social cause. I hope this will cancel the advantage of any single side and lead more often to the resolution of public issues on their merits.

This chapter is divided into three parts. The first part examines the concept of social marketing more closely. The second part distinguishes four types of social causes, each of which is more challenging than the preceding one. The final part describes seven major steps in the social marketing process.

CONCEPT OF SOCIAL MARKETING

The term *social marketing* was first introduced in 1971 to describe the use of marketing principles and techniques to advance a social cause, idea, or behavior (Kotler & Zaltman, 1971). More specifically social marketing is the design, implementation, and control of programs seeking to increase the acceptability of a social idea or cause in a target group. It utilizes concepts from market segmentation, consumer research, concept development, communication, facilitation, incentives, and exchange theory to maximize target group response. Synonymous terms might be *social cause marketing, idea marketing,* or *public issue marketing.*

Four Basic Approaches to Social Change

One can best understand social marketing by seeing it in relationship to the major approaches to producing social change—the legal, technological, economic, and informational approaches. Consider how these approaches apply in inducing people to reduce their cigarette consumption. The legal approach is to pass laws that make cigarette smoking either illegal, costly, or difficult (e.g., prohibiting smoking in public places). The technological approach is to develop an innovation that will help people reduce their smoking or the harm due to smoking (e.g., an antismoking pill, a harmless cigarette). The economic approach is to raise the price or cost of smoking (e.g., higher cigarette taxes, higher insurance rates for smokers). Finally, the informational approach is to direct persuasive information at smokers about the risks of smoking and the advantages of not smoking (e.g., "Warning: The Surgeon General Has Determined That Smoking Is Dangerous to Your Health").

The Emergence and Evolution of Social Marketing

The roots of social marketing are in the informational approach, in the form known as *social advertising.* Many cause groups, struck by the apparent effectiveness of commercial advertising, began to consider its potential for changing public attitudes and behavior. Family planning organizations in India, Sri Lanka, Mexico, and several other countries have sponsored major advertising campaigns attempting to sell people on the idea of having fewer children. Messages on billboards and over radio tell the public that they can have a higher standard of living with fewer children (India) or be happier (Sri Lanka). Nutrition groups have also used advertising extensively to encourage people to adopt better eating habits.

Properly designed, these campaigns can influence attitudes and behavior. The problem is that all too often these campaigns are the only step taken to motivate new behavior, and by themselves, they are usually inadequate. First, the message may be inadequately researched. For example, media campaigns to encourage people in developing countries to improve their diets miss the point that many people lack knowledge of which foods are the most healthful, they may lack the money to buy these goods, and in remote areas, they may not find certain foods available. Second, many people screen out the message through selective perception, distortion, and forgetting. Mass communications have much less direct influence on behavior than has been thought, and much of their influence is mediated through the opinion leadership of other people. Third, many people do not know what to do after their exposure to the message. "Stop smoking—it might kill you" does not help the smoker know how to handle the urge to smoke or where to go for help.

When these limitations were recognized, social advertising evolved into a broader approach known as *social communication.* Much of current social marketing has moved from a narrow advertising approach to a broad social communication/promotion approach to accomplish its objectives. Social communicators make greater use of personal selling and editorial support in addition to mass advertising. Thus, the family planning campaign in India utilizes a network of agents, including doctors, dentists, and barbers, to "talk up" family planning to people with whom they come in contact. Events such as Family Planning Day and family planning fairs, together with buttons, signs, and other media, get the message across.

Only recently has social marketing begun to replace social communication as a larger paradigm for effecting social change. Social marketing adds at least four elements that are missing from a purely social communication approach.

One element is sophisticated *marketing research,* which is used to learn about the market and the probable effectiveness of alternative marketing approaches. Social advertising amounts to a shot in the dark unless it is preceded by careful marketing research. Thus, social marketers concerned with smoking will examine the size of the smoking market, the major market segments and the behavioral characteristics of each, and the cost–benefit impact of targeting different segments and designing appropriate campaigns for each.

The second element added by social marketing is *product development.* Faced with the problem of getting people to stop smoking, a social advertiser or communicator will see the problem largely as one of exhorting people to quit smoking by using health appeals, monetary appeals, or whatever seems appropriate. The social marketer, in addition, will consider existing or potential products that will make it easier for people to adopt the desired behavior, such as guidelines for physicians to use in helping their patients to stop smoking and low-tar and low-nicotine cigarettes. In other words, whenever possible, the social marketer does not stay with the existing product and try to sell it—a sales approach—but rather, searches for the best product to meet the need—a marketing approach.

The third element added by social marketing is the *use of incentives.* Social communicators concentrate on composing messages dramatizing the benefits or disadvantages of different kinds of behaviors. Social marketers go further and design specific incentives to increase the level of motivation. For example, social marketers have advised public health officials who are running immunization campaigns in remote villages to offer small gifts to people who show up for vaccinations. Some hospitals in South America run price specials on certain days in which people who come in for health checkups pay less then the normal charge. The sales promotion area is rich with tools that the marketer can use to promote social causes.

The fourth element added by social marketing is *facilitation.* Since time and effort are necessary investments for anyone wishing to change his or her behavior, marketers consider ways to make it easier for people to adopt the new behavior. For example, smoking cessation classes must be conveniently located and conducted in a professional manner. Marketers are keenly aware of the need to develop convenient and attractive response channels to complement the communication channels. Thus, they are concerned not only with getting people to adopt a new behavior but also with finding ways to facilitate maintenance of the behavior.

Social marketing goes beyond social advertising and social communication in that it involves all "four *p*'s" (product, pricing, placement, and promotion), not just one. Social communicators usually come into the planning process after the objectives, policies, and products have been determined. They have little or no influence on product design, pricing, or distribution. Their job is to promote the organization's objectives and products, using communication media. Social marketers, on the other hand, participate actively in the planning. They advise what products will be acceptable to the target public, what incentives will work best, what distribution systems will be optimal, and what communication program will be effective. They think in exchange terms rather than solely in persuasion terms. They are as interested in improving their offer as they are in modifying the target market's attitude toward the offer. Whereas propagandists take the product, price, and channels as given, social marketers treat them as variables.

Who Does Social Marketing?

Social marketing usually implies that the social marketer is primarily acting in the public interest. Many social causes would be accepted unambiguously as falling under the rubric *social marketing*—for example, civil rights, better nutrition, better health care, and environmental protection movements. There are other causes that are more ambiguous. The marketing of family planning is an example of social marketing but so would be the antimarketing of family planning by religious groups who think it is not in society's interest. Both the protagonists and antagonists of abortion regard their positions to be in the interest of society, and they can plan the marketing of their idea in a social marketing framework. Any social cause or health issue, in fact, can be marketed. We cannot assume, however, that everyone will agree that it is in the public interest (Laczniak, Lusch, & Murphy, 1979).

Social marketing can be carried on by business firms as well as by nonprofit organizations. Consider the following examples.

- Seat belt manufacturers are major supporters of auto safety legislation, partly because they stand to gain.
- Bottled water manufacturers in France have backed efforts to influence French citizens to reduce their alcohol consumption.

- Condom manufacturers have lent support to campaigns against VD because they stand to gain through greater use of condoms.
- Life insurance companies are encouraging people to jog, cut down on fats and sugar, install smoke alarms, and in other ways reduce illness, accidents, and premature deaths, thus cutting insurance claims and raising company profits.

It is clear that business firms sponsor social marketing programs in which they derive a benefit along with the public.

DISTINCTIONS AMONG TYPES OF SOCIAL CAUSES

Social marketing aims to produce an optimal plan for bringing about a desired social change. The fact that the plan is optimal, however, does not guarantee that the target change will be achieved. It depends on how easy or difficult the targeted health change is. Without social marketing thinking, it may be that the desired change has only a 10% chance of being achieved; the best social marketing plan may only increase this probability to 15%. In other words, some changes are relatively easy to effect, even without social marketing; others are supremely difficult to accomplish, even with social marketing.

I will distinguish among four types of health-related changes of increasing difficulty to effect, namely, cognitive change, action change, behavioral change, and value change.

Cognitive Change

There are many health causes that have the limited objective of creating a cognitive change in the target audience. They are called public information or public education campaigns. Many examples can be cited:

- Campaigns to explain the nutritional value of different foods
- Campaigns to expand awareness of Medicare and Medicaid benefits
- Campaigns to bring attention to pressing public health problems, such as those that accompany poverty or pollution

Cognitive change causes seem to be fairly easy to market effectively because they do not seek to change any deep-rooted attitudes or behavior. Their aim is primarily to create awareness or knowledge. The optimal marketing approach would appear to be straightforward. In this case, marketing research would be used to identify the groups that most need the information. Their media habits are identified to serve as guides for distributing and timing effective messages. The messages themselves are formulated on the basis of target audience analysis. They are carried to the audiences through advertising, publicity, personnel, displays, exhibitions, and other means. The effectiveness of the campaign can be measured by postsampling members of the target groups to see how much increase in comprehension has taken place.

Although it may seem that information campaigns should succeed easily, the evidence is quite mixed. Hyman and Sheatsley (1947) give several reasons why information campaigns may fail:

1. There exists a hard core of "chronic know-nothings" who cannot be reached by information campaigns. In fact, "there is something about the uninformed that makes them harder to reach, no matter what the level or nature of the information."
2. The likelihood of being exposed to the information increases with interest in the issue. If few people are initially interested, few will be exposed.
3. The likelihood of being exposed to the information increases with the information compatibility with prior attitudes. People will tend to avoid disagreeable information.
4. People will read different things into the information that they are exposed to, depending on their beliefs and values. The bigot, for example, often does not perceive antiprejudice literature as such. People emerge with a range of different reactions to the same material.

Thus, much thought has to be given to planning the simplest of campaigns—those that are designed to produce cognitive change. The message must be interesting, clear, and consonant with the intended audience values (Douglas, Westley, & Chaffee, 1970).

Action Change

Another class of causes are those attempting to induce a maximum number of persons to take a specific action during a given period. Many examples can be cited:

- Campaigns to attract people to show up for a mass immunization campaign
- Campaigns to attract eligible people to sign up for Medicaid
- Campaigns to attract women over 40 to take annual cancer detection tests
- Campaigns to attract blood donors

Action causes are somewhat harder to market than cognitive change causes. The target market has to comprehend something *and* take specific action based on it. Action involves a cost to the actors. Even if their attitude toward the action is favorable, their carrying it out may be impeded by such factors as distance, time, expense, or plain inertia. For this reason, the marketer has to arrange factors that make it easy for target persons to carry out this action.

Mass immunization campaigns are a good example. Medical teams in Africa visit villages in the hope of inoculating everyone. Over the years a procedure to increase the number of villagers the teams attract has been developed. A marketing team is sent to each village a few weeks before the appearance of the medical team. The marketers meet the village leaders to describe the importance of the program so that the leaders in turn will ask their people to cooperate. The marketers offer monetary or other incentives to the village leaders. They drive a sound truck around the village announcing the date and occasion. They promise rewards to those who show up. Posters are placed in various locations. The medical team arrives when scheduled and uses inoculation equipment that is relatively fast and painless. The whole effect is an orchestration of product, price, place, and promotion—factors that are calculated to achieve the maximum possible turnout.

Behavioral Change

Another class of causes aims to induce or help people change some aspect of their behavior for the sake of their health. Behavioral change causes include the following:

- Efforts to discourage cigarette smoking
- Efforts to discourage excessive consumption of alcohol
- Efforts to discourage the use of hard drugs
- Efforts to help overweight people change their food habits

Behavioral change is harder to achieve than cognitive or one-shot action changes. People must unlearn old habits, learn new habits, and freeze the new pattern of behavior. For example, in the area of birth control, couples have to learn how to use new devices, such as a condom or diaphragm, and get into the habit of using them regularly, without anyone being around to help them or reinforce this behavior. In the area of safe driving, drivers who have a tendency to drink heavily at social gatherings must learn either to drink less or to know when they are not able to drive their own cars. Various campaigns have been directed at problem drivers to condition them to be aware of the problem and the penalties.

Change agents rely primarily on mass communication to influence changes in behavior. In some cases, mass communication can be counterproductive. In the late sixties when many young people were experimenting with hard drugs, advertising agencies, social agencies, and legislators felt that advertising could be a powerful weapon for discouraging hard drug usage. Much money was funded privately and by the government, with donations of time by advertising agencies and media organizations. Fear appeals were first tried, which were followed by informational advertising. Soon some people began to voice doubts about the good that this was doing. UN Secretary General Kurt Waldheim presented a drug evaluation study to the UN in 1972 and cautioned that "special care must be exercised in this connection not to arouse undue curiosity and unwittingly encourage experimentation" ("Wrong Publicity May Push," 1972). Antidrug messages, especially those on television, reach many young people who may never have thought about drugs. These young people do not necessarily perceive the message negatively and might in fact develop a strong curiosity about the subject. This is accompanied by the feeling that if the older generation is spending large amounts of money to talk them out of something, there must be something good in it. They start discussing drugs with their friends and soon learn where to obtain illegal drugs and how to use them. They also learn that drugs are not that dangerous if used carefully. Thus, mass advertising might provoke initial curiosity more than fear and lead the person into exploration and experimentation. The main point is that organizations of individuals often resort to advertising without sufficient knowledge of the audience or without testing the probable effects of their message upon the audience (Ray, Ward, & Lesser, 1973). They fail to create mechanisms that enable people to translate their motivation into appropriate action.

Value Change

The final class of causes attempts to alter deeply felt beliefs or values that a target group holds toward some object or situation. Examples include:

- Efforts to alter people's ideas about abortion
- Efforts to alter people's ideas about the number of children they should have
- Efforts to alter people's ideas about taking blood pressure medication for life

Efforts to change deeply held values are among the most difficult causes to market. People's sense of identity and well-being are rooted in their basic values. Their basic values orient their social, moral, and intellectual perceptions and choices. The intrusion of dissonance into their values creates heavy strain and stress. They will try to avoid dissonant information, rationalize it away, or compartmentalize it so that it does not affect their values. The human psychological system resists information that is disorienting.

Any effort to change people from one basic value orientation to another requires a prolonged and intense program of indoctrination. Even then, it is likely to succeed only to the smallest degree. Consider the classic case of the Chinese indoctrination program for American prisoners of war during the Korean War (Schein, 1956). The circumstances were most propitious for attempting to change the values of a target group. The Chinese had complete control over the informational, physical, and social environment of their captives. Their aim was to alter the beliefs and values of the prisoners toward communism and toward who was to blame for the war. The Chinese suffused their captives with their newspaper and radio propaganda so that the prisoners saw and heard only the Chinese point of view. They divided the prisoners into small groups without their friends and without the normal leadership of officers. They planted spies in the midst of each group to create fear and a lack of trust of other Americans. They lectured endlessly about American war crimes and rewarded the prisoners who gave the slightest positive response. They started with trivial demands for intellectual concession, and as the Americans acceded, they escalated the required responses. They presented photographs and experts as evidence for their point of view. They tailored their techniques to the intelligence, race, and political views of each man. In the end, they succeeded in persuading only 21 prisoners out of tens of thousands to refuse repatriation after the armistice, although many more underwent some alteration of beliefs.

The major factor limiting the success of the Chinese, in spite of their total control over the environment, was that they were a negatively regarded source. Because they were the enemy, the prisoners discounted their credibility. On the other hand, a totalitarian state can be effective if it has the trust of the people. Having control over all the instruments of information and reward, the totalitarian state can undertake to alter the value orientations of its people. Small-group experiments, conducted by Asch, Lewin, and others, confirm the readiness of participants in a group to go along with the group's judgment in spite of their initially resistant opinions (Asch, 1953; Lewin, 1952).

The values that people hold often are pragmatic as well as ideological, making them even more difficult to change. For example, the preference of rural farmers in India for large families makes economic sense. The farmer in his old age has protection in the form of male heirs who will take care of him. Of six children that his wife might bear, only three or four may reach adulthood. Of these, only one or two may be male. Thus, the father thinks in terms of six children to produce a living male heir when he is 65. Furthermore, birth delivery in the rural area costs virtually nothing, and the father can feed his children with scraps of food. At age 6, his child starts running errands, working in the field, or helping the mother, thus being productive. Consequently, when the rural farmer in India hears arguments that he should have fewer children because of overpopulation, it has no meaning for him in his particular life situation. Persuasive communication can have very little impact. In such cases, the state must resort to other measures if it is serious about bringing down the birthrate. Offering a positive economic incentive to have few children may not work because the value of the incentive is usually too small in relation to the value of having another child. The state may try negative economic incentives such as a tax on the number of children, compulsory schooling at the age of 6, which would reduce the productivity of children in rural areas, or a requirement that all children be born in hospitals, which would increase the cost of giving birth. These are harsh measures, but they may become necessary when it becomes clear that the major target groups for family planning—rural families who have many children—are the least likely to change their minds because of persuasive communication.

When values are highly resistant to change, many social planners prefer to use the law to require new behaviors, even if they are not accompanied by attitudinal change. The theory is that, as people have to comply with the new law, forces will be set into motion that will begin to produce the desired attitude change. Consider the case of nonsmoking rules in public buildings. Social attitudes reflecting the acceptance of smoking began to change when rules dictated new nonsmoking behavior. The passage of even a disliked law sets several forces in motion that may accelerate the adoption of the targeted change:

1. The new law helps the law's supporters gain new strength. They coalesce their forces and work harder for its implementation.
2. The new law stimulates more radical proposals, leading citizens to accept the original change in order to ward off the more radical proposals.
3. The new law creates sustained media attention and word-of-mouth discussion that leads people to examine their ideas and values more carefully.
4. The new law elicits conformity on the part of citizens who believe laws are to be obeyed. Conformity eventually leads from mere compliance to acceptance through processes of dissonance reduction.

Thus, when it comes to changing basic attitudes, the most effective means may be to pass laws requiring behavioral conformity, which set forces into motion that may accelerate the acceptance of new values. In this case, the marketer's role is to build a climate favorable to the passage and acceptance of the new law.

THE SOCIAL MARKETING PROCESS

In this final section, we shall describe the major steps in the planning of a social marketing campaign. The steps serve as a review of the marketing process itself. The steps are (1) problem definition, (2) goal setting, (3) target market segmentation, (4) consumer analysis, (5) influence channels analysis, (6) marketing strategy and tactics, and (7) implementation and evaluation. We shall illustrate these steps in connection with the problem of encouraging people to give up or reduce cigarette smoking (Fox & Kotler, 1981).

Problem Definition

For a long time, antismoking groups such as the American Cancer Society and American Heart Association as well as the U.S. surgeon general defined the antismoking problem as that of convincing smokers that cigarette smoking was harmful to their health. Most of the social marketing resources were put into disseminating rational and emotional messages about the harmful effects of smoking. Their success in creating public awareness is clear. A 1975 government-sponsored survey found that between 70% and 80% of current smokers agreed that smoking was harmful to their health (Center for Disease Control, 1976). However, it also became clear that the problem was deeper: Nine out of ten smokers said they would like to quit but found it difficult. In fact, 57% expected to be smoking five years later (Center for Disease Control, 1976). The problem is how to help smokers actually quit smoking—not simply how to convince them to want to stop smoking. Social marketing cannot be effective unless it is addressed to the right problem.

Antismoking forces must begin by researching why smokers start to smoke, why they continue, and why they fail to be able to quit when they want to. A knowledge of the forces that encourage and discourage smoking helps to establish the nature of the problem as well as to suggest intervention strategies. The marketer should examine not only psychological forces but also economic, political, and cultural factors that support and reinforce the smoking habit.

Goal Setting

The social marketers must set measurable goals that they can reasonably hope to accomplish. They might set an overall goal of reducing the number of smokers by 20 million within a 5-year period. They might establish separate goals for each segment of the market. These goals are needed for two reasons. First, they enable the marketers to develop a plan and budget. Second, they establish benchmarks for evaluating the success of the campaign.

Target Market Segmentation

The impact of social marketing efforts is enhanced by target market segmentation. The total population can be divided into nonsmokers, ex-smokers, light smokers, medium smokers, and heavy smokers, on the grounds that each group needs different marketing supports. Each group can be subsegmented by demographic characteristics such as sex, age, socioeconomic status, and place of residence. A further subdivision is possible by using such variables as length of use of cigarettes, motivations for smoking, and readiness to discontinue smoking. Segmentation allows social marketers to do two things: (1) to select specific segments as the focus for their efforts, and (2) to study the behavior of each segment in order to identify the most cost-effective marketing strategies.

Consumer Analysis

Each target market segment needs to be researched in terms of how people think about smoking and what process would be necessary to help them move from their present attitude and behavior to the desired attitudes and behaviors. For example, an important target group is teenage girls, who have shown one of the highest increases of smoking in recent years. An analysis of why teenage girls smoke reveals such factors as a desire to be accepted, to feel grown up, and to reduce tension. Social marketers must try to discover and communicate other ways through which teenage girls can satisfy these same needs.

Influence Channel Analysis

Social marketers need the cooperation of a number of influence channels to carry out their programs. They would like the mass media to donate more public service time to antismoking messages; public schools to put in more effective programs to educate students about the harmfulness of smoking; business establishments to set aside nonsmoking sections; social agencies to establish smokers' clinics; physicians to pass out helping-smokers-quit kits; and legislators to pass new laws. Each target channel must be analyzed with respect to its attitudes and likely responses to various proposals and incentives. Not all channels are equally important, and the social marketers must choose which ones would be the most important to activate.

Social marketing campaigns have to be taken down to the grassroots level—namely, communities. It is often desirable to set up a staff in each community to implement the campaign plan. The workers should have skills in public speaking, preparing written communications, motivating volunteers, and identifying opinion leaders.

At times the social marketing organization may need to bring pressure on certain groups. For example, business establishments such as restaurants may resist establishing separate sections for nonsmokers. They may refuse to talk to the change agents. In this case, a larger view of the influence channel problem is desirable. Figure 1 shows what might be done. The social marketing organization might turn the problem into one of convincing legislators to pass a separate-smoking-section law. To motivate legislators to pass these laws, the organization might first have to influence the general public to support nonsmoking areas in business establish-

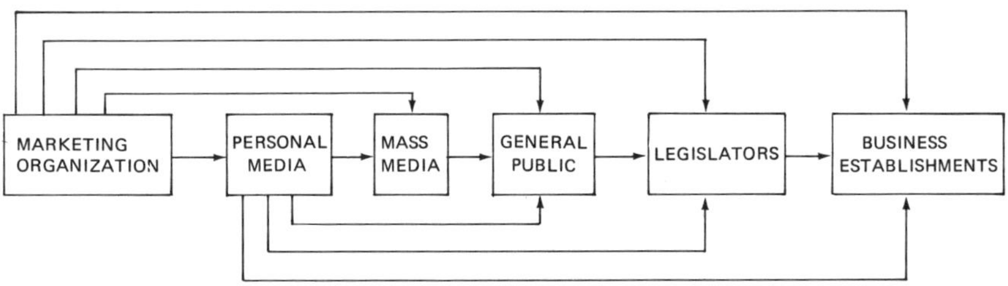

Figure 1. Influence channel analysis.

ments. To reach the general public, mass media would have to be used. To get the mass media to publicize the cause, the marketers would visit editors to sell their cause. Thus, the problem of convincing business establishments to set up separate nonsmoking sections turns out to require an elaborate linking of influence channels.

Marketing Strategies and Tactics

Change agents can now consider possible strategies used by other change agents and generate additional strategies by brainstorming and by reviewing the four *p*'s of the marketing mix. Table 1 shows an application of the four-*p* framework to the problem of discouraging cigarette smoking. Each strategy can be further elaborated. For example, the idea to create a substitute for cigarettes has led to experiments with lettuce leaves as a tobacco substitute. Social marketers would then examine which strategies would be the most cost-effective with which target groups. Choices would

Table 1. Possible Tactics for Countermarketing Smoking

Product
- Require filters on all cigarettes
- Print line on each cigarette as "stop line"
- Make cigarettes shorter
- Sell separately or in individual packs only
- Market water filters or other technology to reduce harmful effects
- Create a substitute for cigarettes

Price
- Raise tax level on cigarettes
- Reduce insurance premiums for nonsmokers, raise for smokers
- Require cigarette companies to contribute to treatment of smoking-related diseases
- Reduce Medicare, Social Security, or other benefits to smokers

Place
- Limit places where cigarettes can be purchased, for example, no sales in food or drug stores, vending machines, PX's, government hospitals
- Limit places where smoking is permitted
- Require registration to purchase cigarettes

Promotion
- Restrict cigarette advertising; for example, no color ads; no pictures, text only; no targeting to new recruits
- Require half of cigarette ad space to present specific health warnings
- Ban all cigarette advertising
- Provide home self-help kits and hot lines
- Broadcast antismoking messages

be made and spelled out in a social marketing plan that would be the basis for developing the necessary budget to wage the campaign. For example, here is what Sweden recently decided to do:

> As illness and death caused by cigarette smoking continue to increase in countries throughout the developing world, Sweden has begun a program that aims to raise a nation of non-smokers, starting with all Swedish children born this year. The program is expected to include intensive anti-smoking education in the schools and in all maternity clinics, progressive restrictions on cigarette advertising and promotion, regular price increases through higher taxation (cigarettes already cost $1.50 a pack in Sweden), prohibitions on smoking in public places and greater efforts to help people who want to stop smoking. (*New York Times,* June 3, 1973)

Program Implementation and Evaluation

The various actions have to be assigned to specific individuals to carry out according to a timetable that is supported by a budget and the controls that would be used to monitor the implementation of the plan and evaluate its effectiveness. Most social marketing plans, unfortunately, are not developed with good evaluation design. Bloom points out that most program administrators are not interested in evaluation research (Bloom, 1980). The thinking of these administrators frequently runs like this:

> We have to spend money on marketing this cause or else Congress (or some other funding agency) won't believe that we're trying to fight the social problem they ordered us to fight. But that doesn't mean that we have to spend any money evaluating marketing. All an evaluation would do is cost us a lot of time, money, and energy without showing us very much. At most, marketing could be shown to have had a weak effect, and a result like this might only get our budget cut. We know our program is accomplishing something. Let's just keep trying our best and not get involved with the hassles and risks of an evaluation study. (Bloom, 1980)

Evaluating the full effects of social marketing campaigns is not an easy task. An effective campaign, such as an antismoking campaign, would have the following attributes:

1. *High incidence of adoption.* A large number of people responded by giving up or reducing their smoking.
2. *High speed of adoption.* Smokers responded to the campaign in a reasonable time.
3. *High continuance of adoption.* A high percentage of those who quit smoking remained nonsmokers for the rest of their lives.
4. *Low cost per unit of successful adoption.* The cost per converted ex-smoker was relatively low.
5. *No major counterproductive consequences.* Ex-smokers did not start suffering from other problems that were worse than smoking.

SUMMARY

Many health professionals are involved in marketing ideas and causes in order to change the behavior of certain groups. Behavior can be changed using legal, technological, economic, and information approaches. The information approach became refined into social advertising and later social communication. Social marketing is a more sophisticated approach that combines informational, economic, and technological approaches. Social marketing is the design, implementation, and control of programs seeking to increase the acceptability of a social idea or cause in a target group. It utilizes concepts of market segmentation, consumer research, concept development, communication, facilitation, incentives, and exchange theory to maximize target group response.

The effectiveness of social marketing techniques will vary with the type of social change being sought. Cognitive change is the most responsive to social marketing. Social marketing may also be effective in producing action change—that is, a particular act. Behavioral change, such as the modification of food, smoking, or drinking habits, is harder to achieve. So is value change, that is, efforts to modify the value orientation of a target market.

The social marketing process consists of the following seven steps: (1) problem definition, (2) goal setting, (3) target market segmentation, (4) consumer analysis, (5) influence channels analysis, (6) marketing strategy and tactics, and (7) implementation and evaluation.

A social marketing approach does not guarantee that the health objectives will be achieved or that the costs will be acceptable. Yet, social marketing appears to represent a bridging mechanism that links the behavioral scientist's knowledge of human behavior with the socially useful implementation of what the knowledge allows. It offers a useful framework for effective health planning at a time when health issues have become more relevant and critical.

REFERENCES

Asch, S. E. Effects of group pressure upon the modification and distortion of judgment. In D. Cartwright & A. Zander (Eds.), *Group dynamics*. New York: Harper & Row, 1953.

Bloom, P. N. Evaluating social marketing programs: Problems and prospects. In *1980 educators' conference proceedings*. Chicago: American Marketing Association, 1980.

Center for Disease Control. *Adult use of tobacco 1975*. Washington, D.C.: Bureau of Health Education, Center for Disease Control, U.S. Public Health Service, June 1976.

Douglas, D. F., Westley, B. H., & Chaffee, S. H. An information campaign that changed community attitudes. *Journalism Quarterly*, Autumn 1970, pp. 479–492.

Fox, K., & Kotler, P. Reducing cigarette smoking: An opportunity for social marketing. *Journal of Health Care Marketing*, January 1981, pp. 8–17.

Hyman, H. H., & Sheatsley, P. B. Some reasons why information campaigns fail. *Public Opinion Quarterly*, 1947, *11*, 412–423.

Kotler, P., & Zaltman, G. Social Marketing: An approach to planned social change. *Journal of Marketing,* July 1971, pp. 3–12.

Laczniak, G. R., Lusch, R. F., & Murphy, P. E. Social marketing: Its ethical dimensions. *Journal of Marketing,* Spring 1979, pp. 29–36.

Lewin, K. Group decision and social change. In T. M. Newcomb & E. L. Hartley (Eds.), *Readings in social psychology.* New York: Holt, Rinehart & Winston, 1952.

Ray, M. L., Ward, S., & Lesser, G. *Experimentation to improve pre-testing of drug abuse education and information campaigns: A summary.* Cambridge, Mass.: Marketing Science Institute, 1973.

Schein, E. H. The Chinese indoctrination program for prisoners of war. *Psychiatry,* May 1956, pp. 149–172.

Sweden aims to forge a nonsmoking nation. *New York Times,* June 3, 1978.

Wrong publicity may push drug use: UN chief. *Chicago Sun Times,* May 8, 1972, p. 30.

3
Analyzing Markets

PATRICK E. MURPHY

Organizations using social marketing techniques in the health field need to understand how to analyze their markets. The essential components of this market analysis are often regarded as the foundations upon which successful marketing programs are built. For example, to meet the needs of potential customers (clients) of a high blood pressure program adequately, some important information about the market must be gathered through research. It is widely known that certain individuals are more susceptible to high blood pressure than others. Through the process of market segmentation, these people can be isolated and a campaign directed toward them.

The purpose of this chapter is to familiarize the reader with marketing research and market segmentation and to give illustrations of how these approaches can be used in a variety of health marketing contexts. Because gathering information about the market for one's product/service should be the initial activity in a marketing program, marketing research is examined first. Several preliminary concerns in undertaking research are identified; the marketing research procedure is explained; and certain related considerations about research are discussed. The notion of market segmentation is then defined; several segmentation variables useful for health marketers are delineated; and the development of a market segmentation strategy is examined. The chapter concludes with a discussion of the importance of research and segmentation in devising an effective social marketing program.

The use of market research and market segmentation is not the exclusive domain of large commercial firms. These techniques should be utilized by all who practice marketing—large or small. As this chapter will point out, there are many

---

PATRICK E. MURPHY • Department of Marketing, Marquette University, Milwaukee, Wisconsin 53233.

inexpensive and relatively simple methods of gathering information about a market. For example, the local health planning agency may have already compiled statistics on the size of various market segments (i.e., elderly, children, percentage of population with heart disease, etc.). Furthermore, it may be possible to conduct some informal research (see exploratory research section) or a small survey very inexpensively.

The hazards of going ahead with any health-related program without adequate market research are many. One possible problem might be that the program would be directed to the wrong market. Second, the potential user of the health service may not fully understand it. Only through research would it be possible to find out if the likely consumers of a stress management course thoroughly understood its components and potential benefits. A third hazard would be the investment of substantial time, energy, and money into a health program without the prospect of recovering at least part of this investment. Finally, the most severe problem is that without marketing research, the demand for the program cannot be accurately estimated. A good example of what might happen is listed in the following quote from a recent article.

> The marketing naivete of the typical hospital is well-illustrated by a hospital in southern Illinois that decided to establish an Adult Day Care Center as a solution to its underutilized space. It designed a whole floor to serve senior citizens who required personal care and services in an ambulatory setting during the day, but who would return home each evening. The cost was $16 a day and transportation was to be provided by the patient's relatives. About the only research that was done on this concept was to note that a lot of elderly people lived within a three-mile radius. The Center was opened with a capacity to handle thirty patients. Only two signed up! (Kotler, 1979, p. 40)

MARKETING RESEARCH

Initial Concerns[1]

Before analyzing the steps of the marketing research procedure and how they relate to health behavior issues, a few initial comments about marketing research are warranted. First, the ultimate objective for engaging in research is to assist decision making by helping to reduce uncertainty. Unless research provides the decision maker with usable information, it is not worth conducting. Second, marketing research should be viewed as necessary throughout an entire social marketing program. Research needs to be conducted before a program begins (i.e., baseline study), during the implementation (i.e., telephone or mail survey asking about the program), and after the project has been completed (i.e., evaluation research). Therefore, it is an ongoing process and not a one-shot affair. Third, a budget should be

[1]Portions of this section were taken from Murphy (1980).

established for research at the inception of the program. This is equally true whether the program is the effort of a single professional or a comprehensive national campaign. In the current era of strict accountability, money spent on research will assist the health professional/administrator in answering questions about how well a particular program met its objectives.

A fourth prerequisite is to define what is meant by marketing research. Specifically, *marketing research* is a systematic process of gathering, analyzing, and interpreting relevant information for decision making. Each of the elements of this definition requires a brief elaboration. A *systematic process* infers that the systems approach is used in the research procedure and that it consists of a series of steps. Initially, specific informational needs must be stated, the information must then be *gathered* by one or several techniques, *analyzed,* and finally *interpreted.* Although much information is available, only that which is *relevant* to the problem at hand needs to be researched. The objective of improved decision making is also made explicit in the definition.

Marketing Research Procedure

Problem Definition/Opportunity Identification

The first, and often most difficult, step in the marketing research procedure is to define the problem concretely or identify the opportunity facing the health care organization (see Table 1). Although it is traditionally thought that research is

Table 1. Marketing Research Procedure

1. Problem definition or opportunity identification
2. Exploratory research
   a. Internal sources
   b. External sources
   c. Secondary sources
3. Sampling plan
   a. Sampling unit specification
   b. Sampling method selection
   c. Sample size determination
4. Questionnaire design
5. Collecting primary data
   a. Observation
   b. Survey—telephone, mail, personal
   c. Experiments
6. Data analysis
   a. Data reduction
   b. Statistical analysis
7. Interpretation and implementation of findings

necessary only when a problem exists, recognition of an opportunity in the marketplace is an equally valid reason for conducting research. A precise problem or opportunity statement at this stage will alleviate many unforeseen difficulties later in the process because it allows the researchers to focus on one manageable issue. The development of this problem or opportunity statement is ideally a collective effort by the administrators, project directors, and researchers. The team approach that has been analyzed for business marketing research might serve as a good model for health care (Locander & Scammell, 1977). The most useful way to discuss this step as it relates to the health field is to provide several illustrations.

Declining attendance at smoking cessation or physical fitness classes or diminishing requests for informational brochures on breast self-examination or high blood pressure should not be viewed as problems. Rather, they are symptoms of underlying problems. These underlying problems may be caused by changes in the marketplace affecting demand for the programs or some element of the marketing mix (product, price, place or channel, and promotion). For example, the physical fitness classes may be held in the summer when there is little demand for them because of other activities (vacations, tennis, boating) taking precedence. It makes sense to measure consumers' attitudes, perceptions, and potential behavior toward a program before introducing it.

The marketing mix factors that the health professional can control may be the source of the problem. For example, the product or service may be too complicated for the consumer to understand. Often, those promoting health-conscious behavior overestimate what the average person will comprehend and do. The staff of the *Stanford Heart Disease Prevention Program* understood that the price in terms of psychological and monetary costs could inhibit the effectiveness of their program. Ignoring or minimizing the intangible costs associated with changes in health behavior is a recurring problem that research can help overcome. The channel of distribution for health-related services may be the source of the problem. If the program is using improper media, the message may never reach the targeted market. The channels available in any community need to be researched adequately before beginning a program. Finally, the promotion of the health program may be directed at too broad a market to be effective. These examples represent only a small sample of possible problems that health practitioners may confront in promoting positive changes in health behavior.

Research should also be conducted when the health practitioners see an opportunity in the environment. For example, certain hospital personnel are recognizing that their facility might be used for meeting community health needs or for preventive health care purposes rather than just for acute care. Specifically, one hospital has developed a headache and stress management clinic, a smoking control program, and a hypertensive patient education program (see Chapter 8 in this volume). Also, Johnson & Johnson perceived an opportunity in developing their *Live for Life* program (see Chapter 7 in this volume). What appear to be opportunities should be researched so that individuals or organizations do not expend large amounts of resources where there is insufficient demand. Finally, it is imperative that the problem or opportunity be adequately identified and defined before moving on to the later stages of the research procedure.

Exploratory Research

The second step in the marketing research procedure (Table 1) is exploratory research. Once the problem or opportunity is defined, the researcher does not immediately begin to collect primary data. Rather, a thorough analysis of the current situation is undertaken. The exploratory research stage encompasses searching informally for information from internal, external, and secondary sources.

Internal sources of information that are useful for conducting preliminary research are administrators, project directors, medical staff members, or anyone within an organization who may have understanding about the program being studied. All potentially informed sources should be consulted in this stage; nothing should be taken for granted. In fact, the person who takes incoming calls may have information about consumers' fears that an individual would not express to the professional staff. Furthermore, internal historical records of attendance at similar programs or the response to a stop-smoking campaign of 5 years ago may potentially contain valuable information relevant to the current situation.

External sources that should be examined for exploratory research purposes include individuals such as consultants, community leaders, or educators who might be familiar with the health program. This effort would be mainly an informal and unscientific poll of these people rather than a comprehensive study. There are two data collection possibilities that could be used in the exploratory research stage.

First, a "thought leader" survey might be conducted using a personal interview format with 10 to 15 community leaders. These leaders would be asked questions about what they perceived to be the significant unmet health care needs of their locality or how a particular program outlining methods to control high blood pressure might have the greatest impact on the community. Examples of specific individuals that could be contacted are major elected officials, chief executives of local businesses, and civic or religious leaders. The thought leaders might provide some rather illuminating observations about certain health organizations or programs.

The second option for gathering informal information from external sources is a "focus group" interview. It consists of several (8 to 12 is ideal) preselected persons being asked a series of in-depth questions by a trained leader (Bellenger & Greenberg, 1978). The focus group usually lasts 1–2 hr and can be held in the evening in a conference room at a convenient location. Group dynamics may lead to responses that individuals would not advance independently. This technique allows the researchers to obtain a thorough understanding of the problem/opportunity being studied. For example, a group of women could be asked to take part in a focus group on information they feel necessary to conduct breast self-examination. If a female leader is used, the participants may express certain fears and lack of knowledge regarding this issue more readily than they would in a more traditional interview format.

The *Comprehensive Health Improvement Program* (CHIP) of Lycoming County, Pennsylvania used both the thought leader study and focus group interviews in planning a mass education intervention program for cardiovascular risk reduction (Greenberg, Saffitz, Gelfand, & Novelli, 1981). Community leaders were consulted about the project that was designed to promote healthy behavior by providing information about smoking, high blood pressure, and serum cholesterol. The focus group interviews were instrumental in helping to create the name CHIP for the program and in designing the campaign logo in the shape of the county.

Secondary sources—the final type of exploratory research—consist of information that was gathered previously and for another purpose but that may be applied to a current context. The U.S. Bureau of the Census contains a multitude of data on individuals and households. On a local level, the chamber of commerce, banks, and newspapers often collect demographic information that they are willing to share. The aforementioned CHIP program used several types of secondary research. Specifically, baseline national health survey data published by the federal government and major corporations "provided representative information on public knowledge, attitudes, and reported practices in regard to many of the health behaviors CHIP is designed to affect" (Greenberg *et al.*, 1981, p. 14). Table 2 shows a list of these surveys. Another valuable secondary source used to gather information on heart disease risk reduction was the National Interaction Retrieval Service (MEDLARS II) of the National Library of Medicine, which provided a comprehensive list of citations for use by CHIP planners. Additional background information for CHIP's mass communication effort was gathered from standard media reference books, and the telephone directory was used to learn more about county resources and services. These illustrations indicate that there is much valuable secondary information available in every community.

Two final points regarding the exploratory research stage need to be stated. First, these sources should be evaluated on the dimensions of relevance, credibility, and accuracy (Enis, 1980). Some information may not be relevant if it was published more than 5 years ago or if it deals with a different area of the country. The credibility of some thought leaders' views might be questioned if certain elected officials were overly optimistic regarding the economic or population growth of the area. Accuracy of a source may be certified by seeking out confirming information.

Second, if this information satisfies these criteria, the research data may sometimes be used to solve the problem or identify the opportunity without further investigation, thus eliminating latter stages of the procedure that are both expensive and time consuming.

Table 2. Major National Health Surveys

Department of Health, Education and Welfare. *Healthy people: The surgeon general's report on health promotion and disease prevention.* Washington, D.C.: U.S. Government Printing Office, DHEW Publication No. (PHS)79-55071, 1979.
Department of Health, Education and Welfare. National Clearinghouse for Smoking and Health. *A survey of physicians, dentists, nurses, pharmacists: Their behavior and attitudes concerning tobacco.* Washington, D.C., 1975.
Department of Health, Education and Welfare. *Diagnosis and management of hypertension: A nationwide survey of physicians' knowledge, attitudes, and reported behavior.* Washington, D.C.: U.S. Government Printing Office, DHEW Publication No. (NIH)79-1056, 1979.
General Mills. *American family report 1978–1979: Family health in an era of stress.* Minneapolis, Minn.: General Mills, 1979.
General Mills. *A summary report on U.S. consumer knowledge, attitudes and practices about nutrition.* Minneapolis, Minn.: General Mills, 1979.
Harris, L., & Associates. *The public and high blood pressure.* Washington, D.C.: DHEW Publication No. (NIH)74-356, 1974.
National High Blood Pressure Education Program. *High blood pressure control: A progress report.* Bethesda, Md., 1979.
Pacific Mutual Life Insurance Company. *Health maintenance survey.* Newport Beach, Cal.: Pacific Mutual Life Insurance Company, 1978.
Perrier Company. *Fitness in America.* New York: Perrier Great Waters of France, Inc., 1979.

Note. From *Planning a Mass Intervention Education for Cardiovascular Risk Reduction: The Case of the Pennsylvania County Health Improvement Program (CHIP)* by R. H. Greenberg, G. B. Saffitz, P. Gelfand, & W. D. Novelli, 1981. Used with permission from the authors.

Sampling Plan

Once it is determined that collection of primary data is necessary (i.e., exploratory research is not sufficient), a sampling plan must be devised. Unless the health practitioner plans to study only a small group such as chief officers for local health organizations, a sample rather than a census is dictated. As indicated in Table 1, there are several specific steps in developing a sampling plan: specification of sampling unit, selection of sampling method, and determination of sample size.

The *sampling unit* refers to who is being studied. It may be a subcultural group such as teenagers, elderly, black males, or middle-aged women. Usually the sampling unit is quite large in number, and only a small percentage of individuals is actually sampled. For health projects carried out in a specific geographic area such as a city or county, census tracks or blocks might be used as sampling units.

A second facet of the sampling plan is the selection of the proper *sampling method.* The most important criterion in sampling is that the sample be representative of the population under consideration. Two major types of sampling procedures may be used—probability and researcher-controlled sampling. Probability sampling draws from the mathematical theory of probability. An example of a random probability sample would be to select individuals who attended a smoking cessation course from a list provided by the sponsor. Stratified homogeneous groups (black males, women under 35, Hispanic teenagers) and cluster geographic area sample (census tracks, zip code areas, city blocks) represent other probability sampling possibilities (Boyd, Westfall, & Stasch, 1977, pp. 336–60).

If the probability sample assumptions cannot be met, nonprobability (researcher-controlled) sampling techniques can be used. Convenience, judgment, and quota sampling are three types of nonprobability sampling (Tull & Hawkins, 1980). Convenience sampling (sampling people on a street corner or using students in a college class) is dangerous because the group may not be representative of the population of interest. Judgment sampling may be used to reach individuals from different socioeconomic areas. For example, the *National High Blood Pressure Education Program* might want to study the reactions of upper-, middle-, and lower-class members to a particular blood pressure control message. Quota sampling may be necessary in certain health-related research when, for example, an investigator wants to study 100 men with high blood pressure. A large number of males may have to be screened, and the sampling would stop when the 100 individuals with high blood pressure were contacted.

The final aspect of the sampling plan is the determination of the desired *sample size.* Naturally, the larger the sample size, the more reliable the conclusions will be. However, trade-offs between the time and money it takes to locate and interview the larger number of respondents must be recognized. This is an especially significant limitation for small practitioner groups or many nonprofit organizations that have limited budgets for this type of research. Members of the mathematics or statistics departments of a local college or university may be consulted by the researcher if sophisticated statistical techniques are to be used to determine the optimal sample size, given certain confidence levels.

Questionnaire Design

While the sampling plan for a research project is being devised, a concurrent activity is questionnaire construction. The process of writing questions that will elicit the needed responses is a difficult process. Any marketing research or social science research text includes a discussion of the important aspects of questionnaire design. The methodology for measuring consumer needs, preferences, perceptions, and satisfaction is beyond the scope of this chapter, but it is discussed in depth elsewhere (Kotler, 1982).

Questionnaires should meet four general criteria. First, the questionnaire should be tailored to the sample being studied. For example, individuals who are familiar with a cancer education project might be asked more in-depth questions about the program than would individuals who are not familiar with the project. Second, the best questionnaires are often the most simple. Ranking or scaling questions should not be used if dichotomous or multiple choice ones will suffice.

Third, the questionnaire should always be pretested on the same types of people (at least 10 people in all) who will be sampled. For instance, if teenagers' attitudes toward smoking are being studied, the questionnaire should be pretested on high-school-age students. Also, during the pretest, the method of administration employed should be identical to that planned for the overall study. Finally, extraneous questions should be eliminated or kept to a minimum. Excessively long questionnaires can tax the patience of the respondents.

Collecting Primary Data

Once the questionnaire is pretested and ready for administration and the sample is drawn, the next step in the research procedure is collection of primary data (see Table 1). There are three major data collection alternatives—observation, survey, and experimentation. Each of these techniques is useful to the health behavior researcher.

As its name implies, *observation* involves watching people's actions or the results of their actions. For example, rather than asking high school students their attitudes or behavior regarding smoking, one might observe what percentage of them light up when they depart from school. The CHIP program made extensive use of observation by touring industrial parks, driving through neighborhoods, riding buses and taxicabs, and visiting bowling alleys and local "hot spots" to learn more about the composition and general attitudes of the people in the area (Greenberg *et al.*, 1981, p. 31).

Unobtrusive measures focus on the results of individuals' behavior rather than the behavior directly and are a special type of observation. The *Stanford Heart Disease Prevention Program* used unobtrusive measures as well as surveys to assess the effects of their mass media campaign. Specifically, they measured aggregate sales of selected food products (e.g., foods high in cholesterol) in local supermarket chains and the use of public physical activity facilities in experimental and control communities. Reduction in sales of targeted foods and increased use of exercise facilities would indicate that the communication campaign had an impact.

In the survey method, researchers ask a predetermined sample questions via telephone or mail or through face-to-face interviews. The telephone is appropriate for a relatively brief questionnaire in a limited geographic area. For example, a telephone survey was used after the airing of the "Heart Health Test" TV special by the Stanford program to gauge the extent of its penetration of the targeted market. Mail surveys are the most common types of surveys. They have the advantage of permitting more in-depth questions because respondents can complete the questionnaire at their leisure. However, their biggest drawback is the low response rate—sometimes 10% or less.

Personal interviews are much more flexible than mail or telephone surveys because the interviewer can rephrase questions and probe for additional information.

Because this method is extremely expensive (often $5 to $10 per interview), health organizations might consider using the personal interview on a limited basis—possibly to verify or more fully understand data gathered by mail or telephone.

Controlled experiments are the final data collection alternative. An experiment is distinctive because cause and effect relationships can be measured (Cox & Enis, 1972). In the commercial world, experiments are set up as test markets for new products. In a test market, a few nationally representative cities are selected as sites for measuring consumer acceptance of new products. The test market approach is beginning to be used by health organizations. The Department of Agriculture recently tested a mass media advertising campaign on nutrition in Madison, Wisconsin and in Knoxville, Tennessee (Dougherty, 1980). Des Moines and Cincinnati served as control cities for the experiment. The impact of print and television advertising and school programs on adults' and children's fruit-eating behavior at snack time was evaluated. Although the results of this campaign are not known, this experiment does represent an illustration of the proper usage of the test market concept. (Also see Chapter 8 in this book for specific experimental manipulations.)

Data Analysis

Once primary data collection is complete, analysis can begin. As shown in Table 1, this usually is a two-step process. First, *data reduction,* which includes getting the data ready for analysis and calculation of descriptive statistics, is performed. Then, *statistical analysis,* which encompasses a more thorough testing of relationships in the data, can be undertaken.

The health behavior researcher must make arrangements for editing, coding, and tabulating the questionnaire as part of the data reduction process. Editing refers to going through the completed questionnaires and making sure they are answered correctly. One important editing issue concerns the trade-off between using open-ended questions versus ones with discrete categories. The open-ended ones are much harder to edit and code, but sometimes the qualitative information gained from these types of questions is worth the extra editing and coding effort. Coding requires establishing categories and assigning data to them. Because most studies with large sample sizes are tabulated by machine, code sheets are used for keypunching to IBM cards or optical scanning. It is essential that this step be taken into account during the questionnaire construction phase and that it be precoded for this purpose. Finally, from the tabulations, a frequency count either in absolute or relative (percentage) terms can be generated. For certain types of surveys, such as awareness of smoking cessation, breast self-examination programs, or promotional efforts to encourage weight loss or increased exercise, this may be a sufficient analysis.

Interpretation and Implementation of Findings

The final step in the marketing research procedure is the interpretation and implementation of the results. This usually requires the preparation of a final written report and often an oral presentation of it. Interpretation of the findings entails drawing conclusions that relate to the initial problem or opportunity and making recommendations from these conclusions. For instance, a possible conclusion from a nutrition information experiment might be that children changed their behavior after exposure to the information but that adults did not. On the basis of these results, the researcher might recommend a target campaign aimed at adults, explicitly stating the benefits of eating fruit as a snack.

The final aspect of the marketing research procedure is implementation. This action is the responsibility of the administrator, and not the researcher, unless they are one and the same. It may not be possible for the administrator to implement the researcher's recommendations because of budgetary or time constraints. Nevertheless, a concrete response to the research results is needed. Implementation is especially important if the health organization is conducting evaluation research on its programs (Bloom & Ford, 1979). If a health behavior program is evaluated, changes called for by the research should be made.

The importance of the implementation phase to the health administrator cannot be overstated. If key administrators work with the researcher in the problem or opportunity-formulation states of the research, they will probably be more apt to react favorably to changes that are an integral part of the implementation process. Research both begins and ends with management.

Related Considerations

Three additional research-related issues should be of concern to those undertaking market research. First, a decision has to be reached about who will actually carry out the research. There is merit in hiring an independent research agency in conducting the actual study. A familiarity with the criteria used in selecting and working with a research agency is needed (Adler, 1975). If only a small, informal, or secondary study is needed, someone within one's own organization may be able to coordinate the project.

A second consideration is the cost of the research. Most grant proposals now require that money be expended for research to evaluate the project. A similar priority should be placed on internally funded programs. In either case, it is important not to underestimate the cost of conducting high-quality research. A comparison of the costs associated with different data collection alternatives should be closely scrutinized. It may be possible to seek the assistance of a local college or university class in conducting research on health promotion. The trade-off between professionalism and the quality of such research should be recognized.

Third, marketing research should be viewed as a tool to facilitate decision making. Research is an aid to administrative decisions, not a substitute for them. For example, the federal or local government might continue to support a high blood pressure educational program for public policy reasons, even if research showed only a moderate level of demand for it. Thus, policy decisions may not always agree with the research results. In most instances, administrators should be guided by the research findings.

MARKET SEGMENTATION

Initial Concerns

The second important aspect of market analysis is *market segmentation.* This notion derives from the diversity of needs expressed by individuals for products and services. Market segmentation refers to the focusing of marketing efforts on a particular group. As some health marketers are learning, they cannot be all things to all people. This section of the chapter will discuss (1) the major variables that can be used to segment a market, and (2) the development of a segmentation strategy for health practitioners.

Market segmentation involves breaking down the total heterogeneous market into smaller, more homogeneous groups that the health practitioner can then profitably satisfy. For instance, if one is developing an awareness campaign for understanding the symptoms of cancer, not all individuals in the United States are going to be equally interested or concerned. Therefore, the market should be subdivided into those smaller groups that may be the most susceptible to the disease. In addition, if the organization cannot serve a particular group realistically, that group does not represent a viable market segment. For example, a small, regional ethnic group that suffers from a rare malady would not be a good market segment for most national health campaigns.

Market Segmentation Variables

Geographic

Individuals from different geographic locations have differing health needs. State, county, and local health organizations obviously practice geographic segmentation. The CHIP program segmented its market initially to one county in Pennsylvania because of the representative nature of its population. The needs of urban versus rural individuals for health programs such as education on exposure to health risks (i.e., chemicals used by farmers versus air pollution in cities) may be very different. The needs of urban inner city inhabitants relative to those in suburban areas need to be delineated as well.

Demographic

The most widely employed type of market segmentation by commercial firms is based on demographics. These are easily identifiable groups, and their size is usually known through census information. For many health change programs, age, sex, income, race or ethnic background, and other demographic variables represent ideal market segments. The much-discussed antismoking public service announcement campaign using Brooke Shields was obviously targeted toward the teenage market ("Lung Unit," 1981; "HHS Scored," 1981). New stress management programs are being instituted to meet the needs of working women. Low-income groups have long been a segment that nutrition-oriented educational efforts have tried to reach. The *National High Blood Pressure Education Program* has prepared brochures specifically directed toward blacks and a Spanish-language program for Latinos. These account for only a small sampling of demographic segmentation activities undertaken by health organizations. This form of segmentation is also applicable on a local or smaller scale level. For example, before a hospital begins a preventive health program for its local community, the 1980 census data, which would reveal the demographic characteristics of that area, should be consulted.

Attitudinal

Attitudinal differences are potentially valuable but less obvious bases for segmentation. If it can be determined through research what percentage of a given group has positive, negative, or neutral attitudes toward changing dietary habits, different messages could be developed for these segments. Those individuals with negative or even neutral attitudes should be given more concrete information about the benefits of the program than those with a positive attitude. A type of attitudinal segmentation was used by the Stanford program in which the stages of hierarchy of effects model (i.e., awareness, comprehension, conviction, action) were applied to a group of smokers. Specifically, they developed messages aimed at those who had already decided to quit smoking in order to encourage the maintenance of their cessation behavior. The most viable method of utilizing attitudinal segmentation is likely to be used in conjunction with demographics because it is often found that certain demographics (age, social class, educational level, etc.) are closely correlated with the attitudes held. Because it is easier to locate and measure these demographic segments, they can sometimes be used as surrogates for attitudinal segmentation.

Behavioral

Another major segmentation variable is an individual's behavior. If behavior can be accurately measured, it can be a superior method of segmentation because it relates to actions rather than attitudes or characteristics of people. All marketers are ultimately concerned with sales (action) or behavior change; therefore behavioral segmentation is a key concept for health providers as well. Two important behavioral segmentation possibilities are life-styles and usage rate. Life-styles refer to the activities, interests, and opinions of individuals. The increasing number of working women and growing emphasis on leisure time are recent life-style developments.

Table 3. Eight Benefit Segments

Segment name	Benefits sought
1. Firefighters	Immediate solution to a problem (pregnancy, breast lump, etc.), shoulder to lean on
2. Desperates	Relief from feeling of desperation, financial stability, marital harmony
3. Worriers	Security about good health, relief from worry
4. Infertiles	Conception, birth, children
5. Married rationals	Freedom of choice, control, financial stability, marital harmony
6. Married—no children	Freedom of choice, financial stability, marital harmony
7. Married—with children	Pregnancy prevention, financial stability, avoid social stigma
8. Singles—without children	Pregnancy prevention to avoid social stigma, retain independence, financial stability

Note. From "The Market for Health Services. Is There a Non-Traditional Consumer?" by G. Miaoulis & J. Bonaguro, *Journal of Health Care Marketing,* 1980–1981, *1,* p. 41. Copyright 1981 by Journal of Health Care Marketing. Reprinted by permission.

Usage rate encompasses how often a product or service is used. The beer industry knows that there is a relatively small segment (20% or less) that consumes the majority of beer (the heavy users).

In Johnson & Johnson's *Live for Life* program, the life-styles of employees are a major factor for use in segmenting them into groups. The nonuser, light-, moderate-, and heavy-user categories can be usefully applied to segmenting individuals into positively related health behaviors (e.g., amount of daily exercise) or negatively related health behaviors (e.g., amount of alcohol consumed, cholesterol intake, stress on the job). It is obvious that different strategies should be employed to affect the behavior of each of the usage-rate groups. Those heavy beer drinkers previously mentioned should be given a message that includes specific problems associated with this consumption level, such as liver problems and the effect of excess weight on heart disease. The moderate alcohol consumer might need only a general message outlining the importance of drinking alcoholic beverages in moderation.

A third behavioral segmentation approach and one of the most intriguing types used by commercial marketers concerns the benefits that consumers are seeking from the purchase of the product or service (Haley, 1968; Myers, 1976). Toothpaste marketers have segmented their market according to benefits of decay prevention, white teeth, and sex appeal. In the health behavior field, the benefits of a longer, more active life from positive behavior change seem obvious. However, these benefits may be too global and too delayed to influence some individuals. Instead, suggesting the financial savings from decreased physicians' or hospital bills through preventive programs, for example, might be a more realistic benefit for underinsured individuals. Table 3 describes eight benefit segments and the benefits sought for a health education agency specializing in birth control and family planning services.

The authors (Miaoulis & Bonaguro, 1980–1981) developed a complete segmentation analysis for each of these groups and a marketing program to reach them. Clearly, a subject for more research is the benefits derived or desired by individuals from certain health behavior programs.

Segmentation Strategy Development

Requirements for Effective Segmentation

To be successful in segmenting a market, three requirements must be met: measurability, accessibility, and substantiality (Kotler, 1984). If it is not possible to identify and measure the size of a potential segment by primary or secondary research, it probably does not represent a viable segment. For instance, the percentage of women who hold an unfavorable attitude toward a breast self-examination education program may be difficult to measure. *Accessibility* refers to how easily a segment can be reached and served. Health programs aimed primarily at residents of rural localities sometimes cannot meet this requirement. *Substantiality* relates to whether a particular segment warrants separate marketing attention. A segment may meet the first two requirements, but conventional marketing wisdom states that if a segment is too small, it should not be served. In the health field, however, a small segment may deserve special treatment because it is a significant social problem in a geographic area.

Target Marketing

Individuals who practice market segmentation can employ three strategies in targeting their marketing program. First, they can decide not to segment the market and to go after the entire markt with one product or service. This is called *undifferentiated* marketing (Kotler, 1984). An example would be a general awareness campaign aimed at all Americans sponsored by the American Cancer Society. As was mentioned previously, most health marketers now realize that an undifferentiated strategy is probably not the optimal one, because the needs of different sections of the market are quite diverse. Therefore, these needs cannot be satisfied with only one campaign or program.

A second strategy entails targeting only a narrow market segment and developing a product or service to meet this group. This is called *concentrated* marketing (Kotler, 1984). Traditionally, foreign auto manufacturers selling their cars in the United States have practiced this strategy (e.g., Mercedez Benz, Honda, Fiat). In the health field, health behavior programs like CHIP and the *Stanford Heart Disease Prevention Program* have concentrated their efforts on certain geographic localities. Because of time and resource limitations, many health professionals are forced to adopt a concentrated strategy.

A third segmentation strategy entails recognizing that the market contains several segments and then developing products or services to meet the needs of the differing groups. This strategy is called *differentiated* marketing (Kotler, 1984). The *National High Blood Pressure Education Program* has recognized that blacks, Latinos, and women represent distinct segments. Therefore, the educational services have been tailored to meet the unique needs of these demographic segments. Differentiated marketing may not take as much time and resources as many health professionals assume. Relatively minor modifications such as showing individuals of differing sex and age in a poster or brochure and tailoring the language of one portion of the program to the specific segment may be adequate. A challenge to marketers trying to change health behavior, therefore, is to determine proper strategies to satisfy the diverse needs of different segments.

Relationship between Research and Segmentation

Marketing research and market segmentation are the essential components of market analysis. It is usually necessary to conduct marketing research to be able to delineate the composition and size of various market segments. However, the research may be of a secondary nature (e.g., census data or published reports), rather than the sometimes expensive primary data collection. Research results, rather than intuitive feelings, should be the cornerstone of developing a market segmentation approach.

Both marketing research and market segmentation should be used with caution by health program decision makers. The tendency of some marketing researchers is to develop a more sophisticated study than is necessary. In the often amorphous area of individuals' attitudes and possible health behavior change, sophisticated analytical techniques and complicated studies should usually be avoided. What is essential is that health program administrators be able to answer basic questions about health-related issues, such as the perceived costs of attending a smoking cessation or stress management course. They should also be able to pinpoint possible target markets.

Market segmentation is sometimes oversold. It is viewed as a panacea to solve the problems of health organizations. Holbert (1979) has listed several limitations to market segmentation studies, including their expense, time-consuming nature, and the fact that they are regarded as a one-shot deal. He also stated that care should be taken that segmentation not turn into fragmentation. In other words, the marketer should not break the market into such small groups that they are meaningless. For instance, different breast self-examination programs should probably not be developed for women in their 40s, 50s, and 60s and older. Health professionals, then, should use segmentation as an important tool to delineate real differences among certain groups, but they should not rely on it as an answer to all problems or look for too fine a distinction among potential consumers.

SUMMARY

This chapter has discussed the use of marketing research and market segmentation as tools for health marketers to employ in analyzing markets better. The chapter began with a definition and explanation of marketing research. The marketing research procedure (Table 1) served as the focus for the discussion of this subject.

The marketing research procedure begins with a definition of a problem or identification of an opportunity that the health practitioner may want to investigate. Exploratory research that entails studying internal, external, and secondary sources is the second step in the procedure. It should be noted that in some instances it is possible to complete the research in this phase. Usually, though, it is necessary to gather primary data. The sampling plan and questionnaire design were identified as integral parts of this process.

Collection of primary data by observation, survey, or experiment was the fifth stage in the marketing research procedure. After the data are collected, data analysis can then begin. The health practitioner was cautioned to use proper statistical procedures in analyzing the data. Finally, the findings of any study must be interpreted, and recommendations of the research team must be implemented. It is the administrator's job to make sure that this implementation occurs or that the reasons for taking no action are conveyed to the researcher.

Market segmentation was the focus of the second half of the chapter. Major market segmentation variables that may be used by health marketers include geographic, demographic (age, sex, income, etc.), attitudinal (positive, negative, and neutral) and behavioral (life-styles, usage rate, and benefits). Once the market is segmented, there are three possible target marketing strategies—undifferentiated, concentrated, and differentiated. Finally, the relationship between research and segmentation was examined, and caveats regarding their proper use were identified.

REFERENCES

Adler, L. How to hire a marketing research agency and working with research agencies. *Sales Management,* November and December 1975, pp. 76–78, 105–107.

Bellenger, D. N., & Greenberg, B. A. *Marketing research: A management information approach.* Homewood, Ill.: Richard D. Irwin, 1978.

Bloom, P. N., & Ford, G. T. Evaluation of consumer education programs. *Journal of Consumer Research,* 1979, *6,* 270–279.

Boyd, H. W., Jr., Westfall, R., & Stasch, S. F. *Marketing research: Text and cases.* Homewood, Ill.: Richard D. Irwin, 1977.

Cox, K. K., & Enis, B. M. *The marketing research process.* Santa Monica, Cal.: Goodyear, 1972.

Dougherty, P. H. Advertising: Spiderman to push nutrition. *The New York Times,* November 7, 1980, D13.

Enis, B. M. *Marketing principles: The management process* (3rd ed.). Santa Monica, Cal.: Goodyear, 1980.

Greenberg, R. H., Saffitz, G. B., Gelfand, P., & Novelli, W. D. *Planning a mass intervention education for cardiovascular risk reduction: The case of the Pennsylvania County Health Improvement Program (CHIP).* Unpublished paper, February 1981. (Available from [Porter, Novelli & Associates, 3240 Prospect Street NW, Washington D.C. 20007])

Haley, R. I. Benefit segmentation: A decision oriented research tool. *Journal of Marketing,* 1968, *32,* 27–33.

HHS scored for snuffing antismoke ads. *Medical World News,* June 22, 1981, p. 25.

Holbert, N. The segmentation trap. *Marketing Review,* May/June 1979, pp. 11–17.

Kotler, P. Strategies for introducing marketing into nonprofit organizations. *Journal of Marketing,* 1979, *43,* 37–44.

Kotler, P. *Marketing management* (5th ed.). Englewood Cliffs, N.J.: Prentice-Hall, 1984.

Kotler, P. Marketing for nonprofit organizations (2nd ed.). Englewood Cliffs, N.J.: Prentice-Hall, 1982.

Locander, W. B., & Scammell, R. W. A team approach to managing the market research process. *MSU Business Topics,* 1977, *25,* 15–26.

Lung unit gets Shields ads. *Advertising Age.* May 18, 1981, p. 107.

Miaoulis, G., & Bonaguro, J. The market for health services: Is there a non-traditional consumer? *Journal of Health Care Marketing,* 1980–1981, *1,* 35–44.

Murphy, P. E. The promises and pitfalls of marketing research in higher education. *Liberal Education,* 1980, *66,* 102–115.

Myers, J. H. Benefit structure analysis: A new tool for product planning. *Journal of Marketing,* October 1976, pp. 23–32.

Tull, D. S., & Hawkins, D. I. *Marketing research: Measurement and method* (2nd ed.). New York: Macmillan, 1980.

4

Developing Marketing Programs

WILLIAM D. NOVELLI

THE POPULARITY OF HEALTH MARKETING

Marketing has been a popular topic among health professionals in recent years. The concept of applying marketing to changing health behaviors among consumers—and professionals—has become almost faddishly popular. A few years ago one health professional said about marketing, "This is just another flash in the pan, like management-by-objectives was a while back. It'll pass." Yet, marketing in the health field is more topical today than ever, and it promises to continue to grow in interest in the foreseeable future.

Conferences have been held on the subject. Papers and articles have been written and presented. Marketing titles have been created in health organizations, and criticisms have been leveled. And all about what? What is marketing? There are textbook definitions, of course. Marketing is said to be based on the concept of *exchange*. It is said to include the four *p*'s (product, price, place, and promotion) in an integrated marketing mix. All true. But the most significant point to be made in defining marketing is that it is a *process* for solving problems. It provides a framework for moving in an orderly, disciplined fashion from *a* to *z*.

Various professions teach and apply problem-solving processes. Accountants have specific, stepped approaches to financial management. Physicians and psychologists move through a process of decision making in patient management. Similarly, marketing professionals have a systematic, data-based process for getting the job done. This orderly approach has appeal in the business world of manufacturing, promoting, selling, and servicing products. It brings discipline to these activities

WILLIAM D. NOVELLI • Porter, Novelli & Associates, 3240 Prospect Street, NW, Washington, D.C. 20007.

and pulls them together into a coherent, manageable whole. It also provides a framework that can be continued beyond the tenure of any single employee or generation of employees. Marketing trainees learn the craft and pass it on. Libraries of marketing plans serve as corporate history. There is continuity.

Marketing companies and their advertising and public relations agencies and research suppliers are very proprietary and secretive about their approaches, their data, and their results. Nevertheless, commercial marketing has become an almost universal discipline with a common language and common techniques. This has come about because of the marketing and advertising trade press, marketing departments in universities with master of business administration programs, conferences and seminars among practitioners, and job switching of marketing professionals. The result is a broad community of marketing people who pursue the same professional objectives and who share knowledge, even though they are usually fiercely competitive with each other. If a Unilever product manager from London meets an account executive from Needham, Harper & Steers in Chicago, the two of them can talk about media buys, product sampling techniques, and 10 second IDs without an interpreter.

Marketing is now being applied to health and other social issues. The same disciplined, stepped approach that makes it appealing in the commercial sector gives it appeal among those who seek to change health behaviors. At this time, it is generally accepted—although critics and doubters still abound—that marketing can be applied to health behavior change.

There are problems, however, in making the leap from marketing goods and services to marketing such behaviors as smoking cessation, therapy maintenance, or breast self-examination. Some of these problems are organizational; it is very difficult to practice marketing in hospitals, institutes, agencies, and voluntary health groups that are structured along nonmarketing lines. The well-managed business sector marketing organization has a marketing person in a key position at the top of the organization chart and numerous well-trained marketing individuals throughout the orgainzation.

Other problems in health marketing center on market analysis. In health settings, there may be little secondary data available about targeted consumers. Moreover, it is difficult to obtain valid, reliable measures of salient aspects of consumer behavior. It is much more difficult, time-consuming, and expensive to probe such health-related issues as sexual activity, family support for cancer patients, and drug abuse as it is to do research related to cake mixes, soft drinks, and cereals. Still more problems arise in dealing with market segmentation, product and pricing strategies, channel selection and use, communications, and evaluation. All these problems combine to make health marketing far more complex and difficult than the commercial marketing of goods and services.

All these problems can be dealt with, to greater or lesser degrees. Marketing *can* be applied to health behavior change. The concepts of exchange, the four *p*'s, and an integrated marketing mix built around consumer wants, needs, and expectations can work in health settings. One problem underlies all the others—a problem that must be addressed first in order that progress can be made in overcoming all the others. It is a problem of *process*.

The framework, the disciplined approach of common marketing techniques that exists in business marketing, does not yet exist in health marketing. There is no universal language, no standard approach, no cadre of well-trained, seasoned health marketing professionals to teach and spread the craft. Many of the people who are learning how to apply marketing in health behavior change are doing so without the benefit of an apprenticeship in a marketing organization. They are health educators, communications and public affairs specialists, social researchers, nurses, administrators, psychologists, and physicians.

Those who do come from marketing backgrounds into the health field must first learn the complexities of the new arena. In addition, they soon find out that commercial marketing techniques cannot simply be applied wholecloth to health. There are many nuances of difference. Examples of these differences are audience segmentation variables, consumer benefits (and barriers), the more limited role of advertising in the overall marketing mix, motivation and utilization of a sales force, intermediary channel strategies, and complexities in research and evaluation.

It will take many more years before marketing in the health field is standardized sufficiently so that a relatively common approach is applied and understood throughout the community of health marketing practitioners and from setting to setting. This process should occur more quickly than it did in commercial marketing, because there are fewer issues of competitive secrecy, confidentiality, and data hording (not to say that these traits are entirely absent).

In the meanwhile, consider the practitioners from several health marketing programs, such as the Family of the Future contraceptive social marketing effort in Cairo, the *National High Blood Pressure Education Program* of the National Institutes of Health, and the marketing program of a large urban hospital. If you were to ask administrators of these programs a single marketing question, such as "What is your process for new product introductions?" you would be likely to hear three different approaches, probably with a liberal smattering of marketing jargon, but with many other medical, health, communications, and social psychology terms tossed in as well, depending on the individual's background. It would be more like speakers of four different Romance languages trying to communicate than if everyone were speaking common language covering a systematic, disciplined, and universal process for health marketing.

The purpose of this chapter is to offer a marketing process for health behavior change. The intent is to bring more order and discipline to the still-new endeavor of health marketing. The ultimate objective, as with all marketing, is to move in an efficient *a*-to-*z* fashion to provide meaningful product benefits in response to consumer needs. The word *meaningful* is important. If the benefits offered are perceived by target consumers to be unimportant, unnecessary, personally irrelevant, or, for some other reason, unappealing or undesirable, the product or service is likely to fail in the marketplace.

The marketing process offered in this chapter is not the only fixed route to follow. Marketing is not—and should not be—a rigid framework. The process here, however, is drawn from successful commercial marketing, adapted to health, and has proved to be workable (with appropriate modifications for differences in product, time, budget, and setting) to a wide variety of health behavior change programs. Although marketing has its share of theory, principles, and hypotheses (as it should if the state of the art is to be advanced), the process put forth is at the practitioner level. Marketing health behavior, like marketing any other set of offerings, must be practical, actionable, cost conscious, and oriented toward results—achieving organizational goals.

THE MARKETING PROCESS

The marketing process is circular, or iterative, with the last stage feeding back into the first in a continuous cycle of replanning and improvement. Another way to think of it is that the action is a spiral. A spiral connotes progress, rather than the idea of going around in a circle. Let us look at a diagram of a workable, easy-to-follow marketing process. It has six steps, which are to be followed in sequence until the process is begun again. The six steps, or stages, are (1) analysis, (2) planning, (3) development, testing, and refining of the plan elements, (4) implementation, (5) assessment of in-market effectiveness, and (6) feedback to Stage 1. The six stages are designed to take into account consumer wants, needs, expectations, and satisfactions/dissatisfactions; formulate program objectives; utilize an integrated marketing

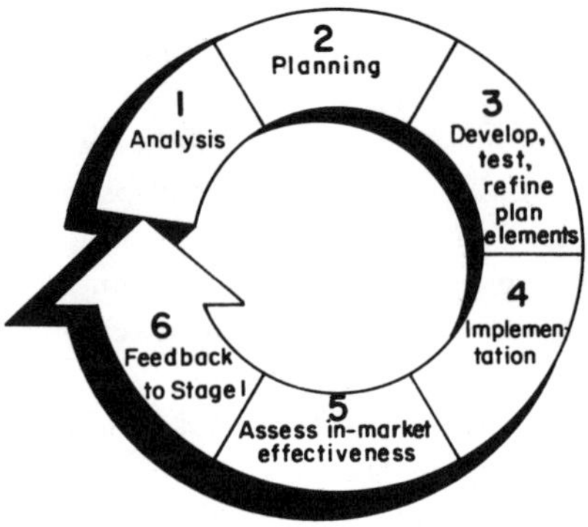

Figure 1. The six stages of the marketing process.

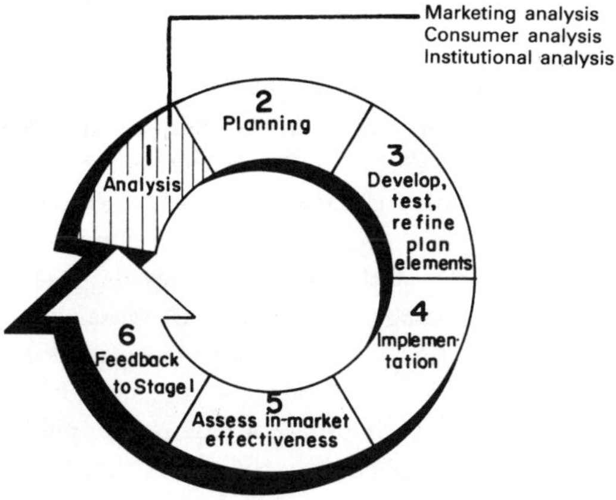

Figure 2. Stage 1 of the marketing process: analysis.

approach and marketing mix (product, price, communication, distribution); and continuously track consumer and market response.

THE FIRST STAGE—ANALYSIS

In this initial step in the marketing process, it is necessary to examine three broad areas: the market, the consumers who make up that market, and the organization and structure within which the health program must operate.

Market Analysis

Defining the market is a good way to begin. In a perfect or totally open marketing situation, you would be looking for large markets, with high levels of consumer demand and reasonably few competitors. If competition is great, you would be searching for areas of competitive vulnerability, either because there appears to be a segment of consumers with unmet needs or because of flaws in the marketing approaches of one or more of the competitors. Thus, you are beginning with the marketplace as the first unit of analysis.

Most health organizations, however, do not operate in such free-flowing ways and cannot simply look for areas of open opportunity. Rather, there must be some early consideration given to organizational mandates and goals. The American Cancer Society, for example, would be prevented by charter, by their board of directors, and by other pressures from moving into the field of controlling muscular dystrophy, even if there appeared to be an expansive market of opportunity there. Thus, market definition is undertaken within the boundaries of the health organization's business. This involves making quantified estimates of the current and future sizes of the market. For an organization interested in smoking cessation, the economic analysis might include the commercial sales, advertising and promotion expenditures, and revenues of the tobacco companies and the Tobacco Institute.[1]

Also, the economic analysis would include expenditures aimed at smoking prevention and cessation. Some of these expenditures are made by consumers to purchase aids (e.g., filters, chewing gum) or clinical assistance (e.g., SmokEnders, voluntary health organization clinics) to cut down or quit smoking. Other expenditures in this antismoking area would include the money spent by national, state, and local agencies and organizations to inform and educate the public about smoking. This information is useful in understanding the trends that are moving within the market and for identifying areas of opportunity where competitive spending may not be dominant.

A second element of market definition is geographical scope. The more precise you can be in identifying the geographic area covered by a program offering, the better the plan will be. Tight geographic market selection makes it easier to focus data collection for planning purposes. In developing a marketing effort for, say, a hospital-based program in northcentral Pennsylvania, try to gather and interpret the economic data for that specific area. A related issue is whether the market being analyzed has any geographic skew. For instance, a national agency looking at the market related to nonemergency surgery would find definite high and low patterns of "consumption" across the country.

Distribution and sales outlets also fall within market definition. It is necessary to know how the current market is structured, because the development of distribution channel strategies will later be an important part of the marketing plan and program. The questions are these: How do current product offerings now *reach* the target consumers? What are the places, or outlets, in which these offerings are exchanged and/or consumed? Take two diverse examples for illustration. The National Cancer Institute (NCI) is charged with improving the behavior of breast cancer detection among the American public and among health professionals. In examining current distribution channels for education efforts directed at asymptomatic women, NCI discovered several instances in which hospitals, largely through the initiative of staff nurses, were teaching breast self-examination (BSE) to inpatients. Based on this early analysis, NCI later included BSE in hospitals as one of its channel strategies in its national plan for information and education on breast cancer.

In a second example, the U.S. Agency for International Development conducted a market analysis prior to assisting the family planning association in

[1]The Tobacco Institute does not sell cigarettes and other tobacco products but does market ideas (e.g., "freedom of choice" to smoke) concerning the growing, manufacture, distribution, promotion, and consumption of these products.

Guatemala in planning a program to market contraceptives through commercial channels in that country. It seemed clear that both the urban and rural Latin populations frequented pharmacies—currently the primary outlet for the sale of commercial contraceptives. However, information was lacking on whether the largely rural Indian groups (about 45% of Guatemala's total population) utilized pharmacies as part of their normal patterns of purchase and consumption. This information is a necessary part of the market analysis for this program, because distribution strategies must be developed for reaching the Indian population via sales outlets that they will accept and use.

A sense of timing is a necessary part of the market definition. Is the market growing or contracting? Are uncontrolled hypertensives increasing or decreasing as part of the total population of those with high blood pressure? Are teenage females a larger market, and at what growth rate, for education and services related to prenatal health? Market trends and growth projections are necessary for planning budgets, interventions, and other aspects of a marketing plan.

A final part of the market analysis is an examination of the resources available for conducting marketing programs within the current structure. Virtually every urban area within the United States contains quality advertising and public relations agencies, distribution firms, colleges and universities (with faculty and departments that include individuals with marketing-related skills), local marketing research companies, and printing and packaging firms. In rural America, however, some of these resources may not exist, and in the Gambia, where the U.S. Agency for International Development (USAID) is testing a program aimed at increasing the practice of oral rehydration for infant diarrhea, it will be necessary to analyze available resources within the market as an almost certain first step for planning ways to supplement local resources.

Consumer Analysis

The second broad area of analysis involves the consumer. In this case, the consumer is the individual in the marketing exchange. In the area of high blood pressure, the ultimate consumer is the hypertensive. However, the analysis might also take into account those who can support and reinforce the hypertensive's therapy behavior. This may also be necessary in marketing efforts in nutrition in which the individual who purchases and prepares the food may be just as important in the exchange as is the person who consumes the food. In other instances, the consumer may be a health professional. In Egypt, efforts to promote interuterine devices (IUDs) to the public must be accompanied by marketing IUDs to pharmacists and physicians, including training programs to teach physicians how to insert the IUDs.

Demographic characteristics are usually the easiest consumer attributes on which to gather data. These attributes might include age, sex, income, education and literacy, social class, family size and life cycle, occupation, religion, race, culture, and ethnicity. Not all these attributes may be relevant to the marketing subject at hand. The more that is known about the consumer population being analyzed, however, the easier it will be to construct a plan to segment, reach, and motivate the target audience ultimately selected for a marketing program. It is also necessary to gather demographic data with which to plan formative and outcome evaluations. A health marketing problem that frequently arises concerns program managers who fail to identify target audiences precisely enough to (1) research the audience further, (2) develop effective offerings and messages, and (3) reach the target effectively and efficiently.

Usually, demographic characteristics of the consumers are important in understanding the current marketplace for planning an effective marketing program. Such health issues as venereal disease, cardiovascular risk reduction, physical fitness, cancer control, innoculation against childhood diseases, family planning, seat belt usage, alcoholism, and nutrition all require demographic target audience analysis.

In addition, geographic attributes of consumers can be important. The region, size of place (e.g., small towns, suburbs, large cities) in which target consumers dwell, population density, climate, and mobility each may be a significant factor in analyzing consumer populations as a prelude to effective marketing planning. In New York State, for instance, geographic attributes are nearly always an important part of initial market analysis because of the dominant role of the New York City market in relation to upstate markets.

The final category of attributes for consumer analysis is psychographic. These attributes include behavioral characteristics. It is far more difficult to collect psychographic data than to assemble demographic and geographic information. Moreover, it is often difficult to figure out how to use psychographic data after they have been collected. However, even if the effort must be a limited one, this part of the consumer analysis can be useful in understanding how, why, and when the market audiences will, or will not, engage in the exchange being planned.

One of the most important psychographic areas involves consumer-reported responses to current marketplace offerings. What do consumers appear to expect? Do they say that they are satisfied or dissatisfied with current offerings, and why? For example, a majority of smokers claim that they would like to stop smoking and that they have made serious attempts to do so in the recent past. Some of these individuals may simply be giving socially acceptable answers because the social acceptability of smoking appears to be on the decline. Those who are genuinely predisposed to quit, however, may constitute a far more susceptible target audience than those who report that they enjoy smoking and expect to continue their behavior. One must also examine the satisfactions and dissatisfactions that those who claim an interest in quitting have had with their past and current quitting efforts. This may result in insights for the development of an offering that appeals to a segment of this audience that desires to stop but has not yet found an offering that meets its needs and expectations.

Other psychographic traits include life-styles and personalities. To cite one example of how these characteristics might affect marketing planning, consider physical fitness. Consumers with long-ingrained sedentary life-styles are probably not prospects for a vigorous aerobic exercise program. They may be more susceptible to an offering that begins slowly, perhaps with leisurely walking, and builds from there.

The benefits that consumers seek are useful attributes of analysis. The Chicago division of the American Cancer Society analyzed female teenage smokers and concluded that the cosmetic benefits of quitting far outweighed the health benefits among this population. Based on this early analysis, the planners went on to devise an information program called *Smoking Stinks,* which featured the benefits of quitting that most appealed to this audience.

User status is another analytical consideration. In some developing nations, women appear to take birth control pills only when their husbands are home from work abroad. Oral contraceptives may not be the best method for this occasional usage, and other methods, such as spermicidal tablets, may be promoted. Seat belt usage is another behavior that may be analyzed on the basis of user status. Individuals may be nonusers, potential users, occasional users, regular users, or ex-users, depending on such factors as length of trip, comfort/discomfort of the device, passengers (e.g., small children), and other influencing factors. Usage *rate* and loyalty status (to the offering and the health behavior *per se*) are related to the user status attribute.

Another important psychographic variable is the readiness stage in which consumers are situated. As is obviously apparent in virtually any health behavior program, consumer populations are not monolithic. Different audience segments are, at any one time, at different stages of consumption and nonconsumption. Marketers sometimes draw the analogy of the leaking bucket in which the water in the bucket is constantly flowing and changing. In the same way, the consumer audience is moving as well. Consumers may move along a continuum: They may be unaware, aware, knowledgeable, interested, ready to buy or try (i.e., exchange); they may be users, or practitioners, and possibly dropouts. The *National High Blood Pressure Education Program* has analyzed this continuum as it relates to hypertension. Researchers in this program have seen a decline in unaware hypertensives and an increase in those aware of their condition. As this occurred, the program staff made strategy adjustments but tried to continue to reach the unaware consumers. Even though this segment is declining, it remains one of the program's target markets.

Finally, media patterns are consumer traits that must be analyzed as part of the psychographic attributes. This is, of course, common practice among health educators, whether or not they are marketing practitioners. There are major differences in media patterns among consumer populations. The better catalogued these patterns, the more effective will be the channel strategies (mass media and interpersonal) that can be planned and executed. Media patterns will become even more complex in the United States as cable and other narrowcasting electronic media become more prevalent.

Institutional Analysis

The third broad area of marketing analysis concerns one's own organization and other institutions and agencies that are directly or indirectly involved in the market. Does the health organization have the financial, management, and staff resources necessary to mount an effective marketing program? If the answer to this analysis is yes, it is still necessary to determine the size and scope of these resources, so that program planning can be scaled to the resources that are available. There are many ways to set marketing budgets and determine program sizes. But it is always prudent to have an initial understanding of the resources available. As one battle-scarred marketing professional with health experience is fond of saying, "Don't plan a champagne party on a beer budget." This is not to say that the small organization or the single practitioner cannot undertake a marketing program. It is, however, important to assess the time, money, and other resources that can be brought to bear realistically.

Equally important to the resources at hand is the organizational commitment that one can expect. Many health organizations are headed by phsyicians and other administrators who see biomedical and clinical research and service delivery as the primary organizational responsibilities. Will they accept health marketing? Will they support it? Sometimes, it may be easier to gain support for the concept than the label. *Marketing* to some health professionals connotes hucksterism, deception, Madison Avenue, or some other negative image. One's first creative assignment may not be consumer message development but the invention of a suitable euphemism for *marketing*.

Part of the organizational commitment must include where in the health organization the marketing effort will be placed. If it is prominently positioned, with access to those who direct the organization and with an opportunity to influence the development of the products (i.e., the health offerings) themselves, then the marketing effort will have a much greater chance for success.

Data gathering and analysis must be seen as precursors to shaping offerings in response to consumer demand and not just for the purposes of deciding how to communicate and distribute offerings that are decreed by other parts of the organization.

The institutional analysis must include an examination of other agencies and organizations in the marketplace in addition to one's own. Analyze both friendly and unfriendly competitors. For example, if one is planning a large-scale smoking cessation program, the tobacco industry is clearly a competitor. But for a hospital planner who is preparing a worksite health promotion program to offer area businesses and industries, similar programs—whether emanating from other hospitals, the YMCA, or the local health department—are competitors to some degree.

Some questions to ask about these organizations include the following:

1. What is the size and scope of their programs?
2. How are their offerings perceived by the target markets? Are they seen as similar or in some way differentiated from one's own?
3. Are there any dissatisfactions among users/acceptors of the competitive offerings?

If you are employed by one of several agencies or organizations working in a health behavior area (e.g., a coalition of groups promoting regional diabetes activities), you must analyze the efforts and activities of the other health organizations that are involved. Friendly competitors can help in many ways, but they can also contribute to fragmented efforts, funding problems, and other difficulties.

Availability of Data

Having identified the areas of analysis to be examined as the first stage in the marketing process, it is useful to discuss how to acquire the necessary data. As an example, consider the *County Health Improvement Program* (CHIP), a 6-year community-based demonstration program in Pennsylvania that seeks to modify behavior related to smoking, high blood pressure, diet, physical inactivity, and obesity. In the absence of data that are specific to the demonstration county, CHIP planners obtained and analyzed national survey data related to each risk factor. These data, sponsored by federal government agencies and by major corporations, provided insights into public perceptions and behaviors and served as backgrounds for a later baseline survey that was conducted to obtain planning and evaluation data that were specific to the project area. In addition, literature searches were conducted on the scientific and epidemiological aspects of heart disease as well as the effective use of mass media and interpersonal communication to bring about health behavior change.

Existing materials and documents containing relevant analytical data were also gathered from government programs and clearinghouses, health agencies, voluntary health organizations, health foundations, and trade associations. The trade associations were identified by using standard references such as the *Encyclopedia of Trade Associations* and *National Trade and Professional Associations*. Standard media reference books were consulted to gather statistics on media outlets, audience coverage and reach, and other media information. Examples of these reference works include

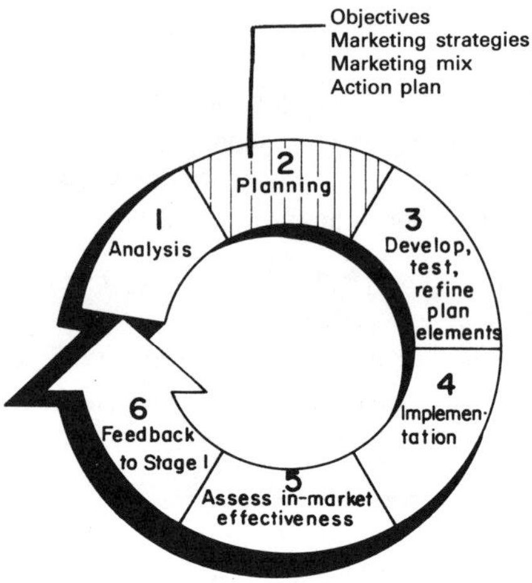

Figure 3. Stage 2 of the marketing process: planning.

Working Press of the Nation, Gebbie Press All-in-One Directory, Standard Rate and Data Service Newspaper Circulation Analysis, Ayers Directory of Publications, Television Fact Book, and *Broadcasting Yearbook.* Media professionals within the geographic market area were also consulted.

Local health organizations, civic groups, church groups, and other community organizations served as sources of information. Thus, both secondary and primary data were utilized. National and regional data were consulted and extrapolated for analysis of the demonstration area. Whenever possible and affordable, local surveys, studies, and inquiries were used to confirm and supplement the larger area data bases.

THE SECOND STAGE—PLANNING

The data collected and analyzed in the first stage now serve as the basis for the second stage—planning. The marketing planning phase includes four broad areas: objectives, marketing strategies, the marketing mix, and an integrated action plan.

The *planning* phase must result in specific blueprints for action. Regardless of the scale of a marketing program, the resources available will be expended in carrying out the plans developed at this point. For smaller programs, this can mean entire budgets and perhaps most available staff and volunteer time. In larger programs, hundreds—perhaps thousands—of hours and dollars will be expended to implement the plans created in this phase. The programs must be clear and viable. A set of plans should be so well conceived and clearly written that they could be followed by another program team that had nothing to do with the analysis or planning stages.

Social and health organizations often lack the competitive pressures that are part of the business world. Managers seldom lose their jobs or gain promotions based on how well the organization does. Consequently, less time and effort goes into formulating plans, and those plans that are turned out are treated as archival rather than action documents. Avoid perfunctory planning. A good plan can be the key to marketing success. It transforms analysis into action, provides consistent direction, identifies milestones for measurement, and sets a unified approach for the entire program management and staff.

Program Structure and Organization

The basic structure of the program must be defined as a first step. This structure will depend on the commitment to the program among organization management. Included with the structure is a clear description of *where* in the organization the marketing effort will be housed. Health marketing is difficult to undertake and is especially difficult in small doses. If the marketing function is out of the organizational mainstream or in a staff support area such as public affairs or public information, results may be limited. This is because the marketing group will have little influence over program (i.e., the product/offering) development and may be restricted primarily to communicating product features, whatever they may be. In this case, the marketing effort would be destined for a mediocre performance from the very beginning.

The question of *who* will undertake the marketing effort within the organization is even more important than the issue of where the marketing program will be placed within the organization. Experienced, capable individuals who can plan and implement good marketing programs are likely to bring greater results, regardless of where and how the organizational boxes are arranged.

There are several options open to a health organization or to practitioners wishing to implement marketing programs. One option is for current managers to purchase marketing services from outside consultants and suppliers. These services might include marketing counsel in planning, services from agencies that specialize in advertising and public relations, and data collection and analysis from research firms. Purchasing such outside services can extend a health organization's marketing skills and manpower without the overhead and related costs of increasing in-house staff.

There are also disadvantages to hiring outside services. Even though this approach may be less costly than increasing organizational staff, outside services can be expensive. Secondly, the skills these outsiders bring to bear may never be mastered by the health organization, and the marketing function will not be institutionalized.

A third disadvantage to the use of commercial advertising and public relations agencies, marketing research suppliers, consultants, and others is that they may lead the health organization astray. Many commercial marketing professionals lack health and social marketing experience. They tend to assume that selling toothpaste or soft drinks is directly analogous to selling health. Often such outsiders appear to rely heavily on the communications aspects of marketing and almost entirely on the mass media. There are two ways to avoid this problem. The first is to choose outside consultants carefully, to be sure they have solid experience in health and social areas. In choosing outside individuals and firms, establish specific selection criteria that can be used throughout the selection phase and for evaluating their on-the-job performance. Set up a screening process at the beginning of your selection process. This will save time and money. Have those who pass the first selection cut write something—preferably a proposal. See how they express themselves and what they have to say.

There is another step in the selection process that is too often ignored, especially by government health agencies with their rigid selection criteria. Go beyond the proposal stage (which is really just a paper competition) to spend time with the people themselves. Talk to the individuals who will actually be doing the marketing work with your health organization. Ask them to take you through the process and the products that they have developed for others. Even if the presentations do not directly parallel your problem, ask yourself if they followed a sound marketing process and a solid course of action.

Ask others about these prospective outside marketing support firms and individuals. Do not just speak to their current clients because these people are apt to be overly flattering. Afterall, if current clients give you a negative reference, it makes the client look a little silly for continuing the relationship. Therefore, it is also wise to gather references from *former* clients. They may provide a different perspective.

A second option open to a health organization wishing to implement marketing programs is to establish an internal marketing services department to develop and implement health programs and to serve as support staff for other departments in the organization. An internal marketing group should begin with a marketing director who has broad marketing experience, including the marketing of health-related offerings. The more highly placed the marketing director is within the overall health organizational hierarchy, the more effective the marketing group is likely to be.

Following the marketing director, the next most important job is probably the director of marketing research. If only these two individuals are in place, the internal marketing unit should be able to operate effectively at establishing marketing direction, managing and overseeing outside consultants and suppliers, anticipating social, political, economic, and organizational trends that affect the organization's marketing efforts, and evaluating results.

If budget and scope permit, the next internal marketing role to fill would be that of the director of marketing communications. This assumes that the marketing department is operating as an autonomous unit and is not folded into the organization's public affairs, public relations, or public information department. In most health organizations, there is some sort of communications structure, and any marketing efforts are housed there. A few organizations have reversed this pattern. The United Way of America has what essentially is a marketing-oriented department (although it has a communications title!), and various communications functions (e.g., public relations, advertising) are subsumed within it.

In setting up an internal marketing staff within a health organization, it is necessary to recognize that marketing is the newcomer and must fit compatibly into the organizational structure. Health agencies and institutions are not likely to reorganize totally and emerge as marketing structures.

Even if an internal marketing services department is created, outside suppliers are likely to be needed. An important organizational role of the internal department is to serve as a good client to the outside consultants and suppliers. Patience is necessary to educate the outside members of the team and to listen to their questions, ideas, and concerns. Their suggestions may or may not be brilliant strategies or breakthrough ideas, but they do come from a different perspective than one's own, and you are paying for them. Being a good client also requires close involvement and reasonable decision-making authority. The key is to find the delicate balance between too much supervision that will smother your outside consultants and too much leeway that will result in superficial, disappointing results.

Setting Marketing Program Objectives

Once the marketing structure is set and the organizational goals are clear, one must identify specific marketing objectives. This is not easy to do. First, the marketing objectives must be realistic. It is tempting to overstate, or overpromise, objectives that call for health behavior change. Most health behavior change programs—whether or not marketing techniques were utilized—have not succeeded in the long term. Problems have included an overreliance on mass media, insufficient program resources, lack of continuity, single rather than multiple approaches and channels, and insufficient research. Most of these difficulties began with objectives that were too ambitious, too broad, and too difficult to translate into action.

In addition to being realistic, marketing objectives must be set in priority. Not all objectives are equally important. Some must preceed others. Moreover, most health organizations have restricted budgets, which necessitates setting priorities for a given set of objectives.

Program corrections must often be made in the course of implementation phases. To plan these corrections and to assess overall progress, it is necessary to quantify objectives to the extent possible in early stages of planning. An objective calling for an increase in the number of identified hypertensives within a given geographic area would be more useful if the percentage of anticipated increase was stated. This requires a data base that indicates current levels of identified hypertensives and a realistic estimate of what can be accomplished in terms of increase. If objectives are not quantified, it becomes difficult, if not impossible, to monitor and evaluate the effort realistically.

Finally, marketing objectives must be consistent over time. Consistency is necessary in virtually any marketing effort, but is especially so in social and health change programs. Health programs that vary their objectives frequently may disrupt the continuity needed to move health consumers beyond awareness and interest to a point of behavioral trial, acceptance, and maintenance.

Market Target Segmentation

Much has been written in this book (see Chapter 3) and in other volumes about social marketing segmentation. Rather than reiterate the steps and characteristics involved in segmentation, this section will stress the necessity of segmentation. Health-consumer populations are seldom, if ever, monolithic. Men differ from women in selective exposure to health messages and in acceptance of personal susceptibility. Younger individuals sometimes respond to different health appeals than do older consumers. Risk factors, benefits sought, life-styles, and other factors vary from one population segment to another. To market health effectively, it is necessary to isoate high-priority segments and to tailor the marketing program for each segment. Undifferentiated marketing—that is, treating all consumers the same way—ignores the basic differences among clusters of target populations and lessens opportunities for success.

Marketing Entry

Part of strategy development is to determine exactly how a health organization or practitioner will move into a particular market. One strategy is acquisition, in which a product or offering is acquired from another place. For example, the American Hospital Association offers programs that individual hospitals can provide to corporations in response to the growing demand for health promotion in worksettings. Another strategy for entering a market is collaboration with other organizations or individuals. To cite one example, the American Dental Association collaborated with the National Cancer Institute to develop, promote, and evaluate a program to teach smoking cessation skills to dental patients. A final entry strategy is internal development and introduction, in which a health organization applies its own resources and skills to plan, implement, and evaluate marketing programs.

Marketing Mix Strategies

Once objectives have been set and audiences segmented, one can devise strategies for each element in the marketing mix. By *marketing mix* is meant a combination of the four *p*'s that make up the essential elements of a marketing effort.

Product

Product refers to the offering that is exchanged with the consumer for a price. In health, the product, or offering, may be a tangible good (e.g., a book on fitness or an exercise cycle), a service (e.g., insurance or health risk assessment), an idea (e.g., self-care or disease prevention) or a practice (seat belt usage or reduced alcohol consumption).

Price

When products are sold, the consumer usually exchanges money for a given product or service and the benefits it provides. In health marketing, there can also be money involved, such as a fee for counseling services, but other prices may be charged as well, such as time and inconvenience (e.g., waiting 4 hr for a 3-minute lab test), psychic prices (e.g., facing social disapproval among adolescent peers for refusing to experiment with drugs), and physical prices (e.g., weight gain associated with quitting smoking).

Place

Place refers to the channels by which the product reaches target consumers and/or the place in which it is offered (e.g., the classroom, the pharmacy, the hospital).

Promotion

Promotion refers to the communication aspects of a marketing program and may involve advertising (paid or public service), publicity, personal contact, and various other promotion approaches (e.g., package inserts, point-of-decision materials, sandwich boards, T shirts with messages).

The first element of the marketing mix to consider is the product. An important strategy decision concerns product *positioning.* This involves a careful study of market segments in order to select a viable niche in the marketplace for the product and to position the product (e.g., an exercise program) at some point on the spectrum of what the audience segment wants and in relation to where competitive offerings are located. Assume that the category of working women aged 34–49 is a prime segment for an exercise program. Assume further that research among this segment indicates that demand is for a moderate exercise approach combined with stress reduction and weight control. Before positioning the product to meet this demand, it is necessary to look at one additional factor—competition. If several other programs are similar in scope and are aimed at the same consumer segment, it will be necessary to decide whether to meet the competition head on or to seek another positioning or place in the product spectrum where there is less competition.

Other product strategy decisions involve carefully selecting appropriate characteristics for the offering. One useful way to look at a health product is in terms of performance characteristics and perception characteristics. As an example, consider the introduction of a new oral contraceptive into the marketplace in a developing country. *Performance characteristics* are those attributes that relate to the product's efficacy. *Perception characteristics* do not directly relate to how well the product works, but they do provide signals about the product that influence consumer acceptance. Such attributes as color of the pills, package design, and product name are examples of perception characteristics. There may be some attributes of an oral contraceptive, such as usage instructions, that overlap both performance and perception.

Distribution strategies are also part of planning the marketing mix. The means of disseminating the offering to targeted consumers must be identified. The distribution may be direct from the health organization to the ultimate consumer. For instance the *Reach to Recovery* program of the American Cancer Society (ACS) is designed to provide services and information directly from ACS volunteers to mastectomy patients. In other cases, such as the *National High Blood Pressure Education Program,* offerings are designed to be delivered to consumers through intermediaries, such as state- and community-based hypertension programs.

Another part of distribution strategy development is to determine the place at which the program will be available to the target market. In offering smoking prevention programs to adolescents, schools are obvious places for the offering. But other places (e.g., Boys' Clubs, YMCAs, sports facilities) may also be considered.

Perhaps the most difficult strategies to develop in health programs relate to price. In marketing good health, the development of a pricing strategy usually involves efforts to reduce the monetary, psychic, energy, and time costs incurred by consumers when engaging in the desired social behavior. An example of a *monetary* price that the health consumer must pay is the expense of filling a prescription for medication. A *psychic* price example is the cost to a preteen of saying "no" to cigarettes or drugs in the face of peer pressure. The Lung Association of Maryland has developed a curriculum module called *Smoking Deserves a Smart Answer,* which uses humor as a way for fifth-grade students to reduce the price of peer influence. Health consumers pay prices in terms of energy, or effort, as in getting to and from a weight reduction counseling program or in carrying out intensive mastectomy rehabilitation exercises.

The price of time that health consumers must pay to engage in a desired behavior works two ways. First, there is time expended. As an irate patient once wrote, "Two weeks ago I waited four hours for a test taking three minutes to administer. If I don't wait in my lawyer's office, why must I wait in my doctor's?" The other side of the time issue is opportunity costs. That is, what opportunities are foregone to the consumer who spends time undertaking a recommended healthful practice? Two investigators (Fine, 1981; Fox, 1980) have developed social pricing strategies in a social marketing context, and both view attention to price as an essential step in the exchange process.

The fourth element in developing marketing mix strategies, after product, distribution, and price, is the communication strategy. As with the other strategies in the mix, this strategy statement is based on the earlier stage of analysis. The communication strategy should contain

1. the basic *benefits* that the target consumer can expect (e.g., longer, healthier life, a return to normal life-style activities, fewer cavities);
2. *reasons why* the consumer can or should believe the offering (e.g., the health behavior) will work and will provide the promised benefits (e.g., "thousands of men and women have already quit smoking using this proven approach," or "scientific studies show . . .");
3. *specific action* the consumer is expected to undertake (e.g., "call this toll-free number" or "take the salt shaker off the table"); and
4. the *tone* or *image* to be conveyed over time (e.g., upbeat and optimistic, serious, medical, scientific).

The purpose of this strategy is to establish long-term continuity for communication and to provide guidance and direction for creative message development. Moreover, the strategy should also serve as a reference for measuring communication. For instance, if the major benefit in the strategy is increased self-esteem related to fitness, then message testing should reveal how well this specific benefit was communicated.

An effective communication strategy should be clear and simple, with a minimum of ideas and directions, and devoid of executional considerations. The strategy statement, in other words, should deal only with *what* is to be communicated, not *how* to do so. For example, it should not include directions on the length of messages or the media to be used, nor should it include suggestions on use of, say, animated characters, physicians, or celebrities as spokespersons. These executional devices are brought in later, during message development. At this point, they could cloud the issue and obstruct expressing the benefits on which the product appeal must hinge.

In addition to the strategy statement, other parts of the communication component should include tactical considerations.

1. Mass media. Identify the media that will be used and the weight that will be given to each in terms of budget and effort, the approaches that will be

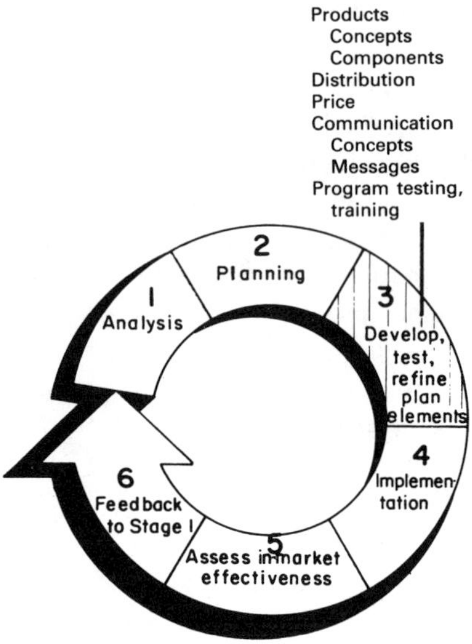

Figure 4. Stage 3 of the marketing process: development, testing, and refinement of plan elements.

taken (e.g., publicity, paid and/or public service advertising) and the timing (e.g., continuous, steady level, periodic bursts or flights, heavy introductory phase followed by lower sustaining levels).

2. Interpersonal channels. This component should be integrated with the distribution strategy, especially if intermediary or middlemen approaches are planned, such as community organizations, opinion leaders, a sales force, or professional associations. Other interpersonal considerations include promotions, point of decision (e.g., supermarket or cafeteria nutrition displays), trade shows, conference exhibits, rallies, and other events.

When all of this planning is accomplished and reviews and approvals are complete, the final step in this stage of the marketing process model is to integrate all components into a single action plan. This plan is the blueprint for everything that follows. It incorporates all preceding elements and includes schedules, milestones in terms of process measures (e.g., levels of awareness, trial, adoption, numbers of brochures distributed, prescriptions filled), outcome measures, a total marketing budget, and a budget and schedule for each element in the marketing mix.

In the private sector, this action plan usually is referred to every day. It is arrived at only after considerable effort and review. Now it guides all that follows. The same attention must be paid to the action plan in a health marketing effort. It must not gather dust on a shelf. It represents an already considerable investment and the best thinking that could be brought to bear. Now it must be a road map for development, implementation, and assessment.

THE THIRD STAGE—DEVELOPMENT, TESTING, AND REFINEMENT OF PLAN ELEMENTS

The first steps in executing the action plan occur in Stage 3 of the marketing process. Here, the elements of the marketing mix (i.e., product, distribution, price, and communication) are developed and tested, and the program is refined.

The initial step in this stage is product concept development and testing. This is a step often overlooked or abbreviated in health marketing, to the detriment of the eventual program. Product concepts stem from the marketing mix strategies that were outlined in Stage 2—planning—and these in turn were predicated on the market, consumer, and institutional analysis performed in Stage 1.

The product in a health program may be tangible or intangible. Much has been written about the notion of product in a social and health context. Several texts (Fine, 1981; Kotler, 1982) are especially useful. The product concept is the underlying idea for positioning new products or repositioning established ones in relation to target market wants, needs, and expectations.

In the commercial products field, a product concept might be the following:

> A hair conditioner that keeps your hair looking beautiful all the time, because you can use it anytime—when you shampoo and between shampoos.

In developing a family planning program for a developing nation, consumer, market and institutional analysis, and product strategy development might lead to this example of a health product concept:

> A contraceptive for women that you use only when you are having intercourse—no insertions by a doctor, no injections, and no side effects.

There is no question that complex health behaviors that must be maintained over considerable periods of time make it difficult to formulate a simple, meaningful product concept around which a marketing program can be built. But this is all the more reason to formulate and test product concepts carefully before full program development. Testing at this stage is usually on a small scale and is designed to determine market interest and to remedy any weaknesses that are uncovered.

A second aspect of product development is to create and test product components. Product components include package designs, sizes, instructions, colors, textures, shapes, dosages, fragrances, disposability, refills, and ability to be recycled. These product components, as stated earlier, may relate to the performance characteristics of the product, the perception characteristics, or to both. In either case, they may influence trial, adoption, and maintenance or continued usage by the target market.

Distribution elements may also be examined at this point. The channels of distribution as well as point-of-use or purchase outlets may be pilot tested. For instance, a pharmaceutical company agreed to have its detail force distribute a book on breast cancer developed by the National Cancer Institute (NCI) for physicians (and other health professionals). NCI wanted a preliminary assessment of this channel of distribution to determine how it would be perceived by physicians when compared to other channels such as direct mail.

An example of a point-of-sale or purchase outlet is a program in Egypt that markets IUDs through pharmacies. An early-stage issue was how consumers would perceive this approach and whether they would take the purchased IUD to a referred physician for insertion. An equally important consideration was how physicians would view pharmacies as a distribution outlet for this product.

It is difficult to assess pricing strategies at this early point. Usually, it is more helpful to wait until the prototype evaluation and test market steps, which are described later in this stage, are utilized. In commercial marketing and health marketing, however, price is sometimes assessed as part of product concept development and testing. For example, in the concept for a hair conditioner described earlier that "keeps your hair looking beautiful all the time," a monetary price may be attached to the concept to gauge consumer perceptions of product value. In a health example, in testing product concepts concerning smoking cessation clinics designed especially for nurses, a monetary price for attending the classes was included in the concept to provide a more realistic appraisal of interest in the offering.

Communication concepts and messages are also developed and tested during this stage. Communication concepts are based on the communication strategy (the benefits, reasons why, specific action the consumer should undertake, and the tone) and contain ideas for a full message. Concepts may consist of rough art, words and phrases and may include a key summary line. These key summary lines are also referred to as key selling statements or promise lines. They help to bring vitality to the strategy, to make the concept memorable and perhaps provocative. Consider the examples of products/offerings, with their strategy benefits and summary lines in Table 1.

Pretesting concepts at this stage can provide direction for eliminating weaker approaches and identifying message concepts that appear to have the most potential. Sometimes variations, or entirely new concepts, emerge from respondent reactions.

Once the concepts (often with summary or promise lines) with the most potential have been prepared, pretested, and refined, entire messages can then be created. These may be full radio announcements, booklets, posters, transportation placards, television spots, or other vehicles.

These messages should be produced in rough form, for pretesting and refinement, if warranted, before the expense and commitment of final production. The pretesting is necessary to assess comprehension, estimate message recall, identify strong and weak points in the message, assess personal relevance to the market

Table 1. Examples of Offerings with Their Strategy Benefits and Summary Lines

Offering	Benefit	Summary line
Dial soap	Social reassurance	"Aren't you glad you use Dial? Don't you wish everyone did?"
Food stamps[a]	Honest assistance, no stigma	"Food stamps—not a handout, just a hand."
Midas muffler	Expertise vs. neighborhood gas stations	"At Midas we're specialists. We have to do a better job."
High blood pressure control[b]	Self- and family protection	"Do it for yourself, and all the loved ones in your life."

[a]From a 1979 program in New York State to communicate revised enrollment requirements and attract eligible recipients.
[b]*National High Blood Pressure Education Program,* National Heart, Lung, and Blood Institute.

target, and gauge sensitive or controversial aspects of the message that may require revision. *Pretesting in Health Communications,* published by the National Cancer Institute (1982), is an excellent guidebook with approaches and numerous examples for assessing and improving health messages and materials.

The booklet describes seven methods of concept and message pretesting.

1. Readability testing is a simple pretesting technique using readability formulas (no test respondents are required) to predict the reading-comprehension level a person must have in order to understand written materials.
2. Focus group interviews are a form of qualitative (not statistically projectable, but diagnostic in nature) research used to obtain insights into target audience perceptions, beliefs, and language in the early stages of health communication development.
3. Individual in-depth interviews are also qualitative, but they utilize individual, rather than group, responses. They are used to assess comprehension as well as feelings, emotions, attitudes, and prejudices.
4. Central location intercept interviews station interviewers at a point frequented by individuals from desired target audiences (e.g., a mall to reach women with preschool children, a beach area to reach those at risk to melanoma). They are not statistically representative of an entire target population, but central location samples are larger than those used in focus groups or in-depth interviews.
5. Self-administered questionnaires can be mailed or handed to respondents along with test materials (e.g., a programmed learning booklet on weight control). This can be a useful technique when the individual must take time to review the test materials and when a health organization or practitioner has limited resources.

6. Health Message Testing Service is a standard system of pretesting health public service announcements for radio and television, which assesses individual messages and also compares them to normative scores based on compilations of data from many health message tests.
7. Gatekeeper review refers to assessments of materials by health professionals, the media, and other intermediaries through whom some messages must pass if they are to reach ultimate consumer target audiences. They are usually conducted simultaneously with audience pretesting so that data from both groups can be analyzed to provide direction for possible revisions.

In concept and message pretesting, it is important to utilize respondents drawn from the specific segments identified in the plan as the target markets. It is far less useful to test among a general audience, although in most cases this may be better than to conduct no testing at all.

Once these steps have been taken to develop and pretest product, distribution, pricing, and communication elements, the next series of steps in Stage 3 may be undertaken. These are concerned with *program refinement*. The three steps of program refinement are *prototype evaluation, full-scale test market,* and *regional distribution.* A fourth aspect at this point is *training* of the sales force, intermediary organizations, distribution firms (if involved), and necessary support personnel.

Prototype evaluation consists of assembling all components of the program in a form as close as possible to its final form and obtaining a realistic assessment of market reaction. In this way, changes may be made before more extensive, more costly steps are undertaken. It may not be possible to shape the program exactly as it would later appear in a finished form in the marketplace. For example, in a small-scale prototype evaluation, mass communications may not be feasible and would have to be simulated in some way.

Here are two examples of prototype evaluations.

- A new product—oral pills—is being added to the product line of Family of the Future, a contraceptive marketing organization in Cairo, Alexandria, and other urban areas in Egypt. Following the development of a market segmentation plan and product positioning and after the selection of a name, a message approach, packaging, and instructions, the product will undergo a prototype assessment. A panel of users (new users and women who have discontinued use of other orals) will be asked to use the product for several months (i.e., product cycles). Consumer reaction to the product (e.g., message, name, packaging, instructions, efficacy, side effects, user and partner satisfactions/dissatisfactions) will be assessed.

- The American Pharmaceutical Association and the National Cancer Institute (APhA/NCI) are developing a program to encourage and equip pharmacists to educate patients about interaction of cigarette smoking and medication and to teach skills and reinforce patients who want to quit smoking. The program, in prototype form, was tested at 20 pharmacies—10 in Baltimore and 10 in Los Angeles—with pharmacists who were specially recruited for the prototype evaluation.

In both examples, some compromises will have to be made in simulating the full programs. However, sufficient realism will exist, and sufficient feedback will be gained to make revisions, if necessary, in the program components before proceeding to the next level—a full-scale test market. In the test market stage, a larger, more realistic assessment is possible. For instance, the Family of the Future may expand from its prototype test among a panel of users to a test market in the city of Alexandria, Egypt. The APhA/NCI program may move from a prototype effort among 20 specially recruited pharmacies to encompass an entire state, with urban and rural settings. Perhaps two variations of the program will be developed, with one applied to Baltimore and the other to Los Angeles. Control markets may also be necessary.

The next expansion of the program may be that of a regional distribution. Although not always necessary or affordable in terms of time or budget, a regional distribution is the best indication of how the program will fare in full, national distribution. If the program being developed is for a smaller geographic area (e.g., a county or state), the same approach of prototype assessment/test market(s)/regional distribution can be applied but on a scale appropriate to the program size.

Just as larger organizations conduct prototype, test market, and regional assessments, an organization or practitioner in a single community or single location can undertake similar stepped approaches before full implementation. A hospital could test a wellness program among one corporation before expanding. The YMCA might pilot test a moderate aerobics program for older persons in one Y before going citywide. A dentist might distribute information on prepayment programs to a

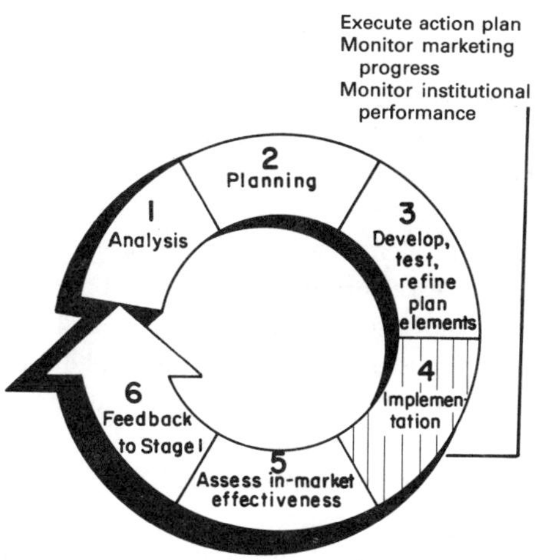

Figure 5. Stage 4 of the marketing process: implementation.

sample of his or her patients before investing more of his or her resources in a broader effort.

At some point in this process of program refinement, it is usually necessary to prepare training materials and conduct training sessions for the middlemen involved in the program. In health programs, these may be medical professionals, civic/social organizations, government staff (federal, state, county, or local), actual wholesale distributors (as in the example of the Egyptian contraceptive program), or other intermediaries. This training, like the other program components, can be refined and expanded as more is learned at each level of development.

THE FOURTH STAGE—IMPLEMENTATION

At this point in the marketing process, the full program is put into effect. This requires implementing the plan of action prepared in Stage 2, monitoring marketing progress, and monitoring the institutional/structural performance of the health marketing organization.

In implementing the plan of action, the full expansion, or "rollout," of the program is undertaken, from whatever level of testing was last employed (prototype, full-scale test market, or regional distribution). This is a critical point in the marketing process. It is the least creative or analytical and for that reason may be delegated to junior staff or otherwise receive less management attention than the previous steps. Yet the details and logistics control of this implementation are central to the success of the entire program. The most well-conceived and well-designed health programs will fail if they are not properly put into place so that they can work.

As part of this plan execution, the communication elements—advertising, publicity, interpersonal channels, promotion, and point of purchase/point of decision—must be activated. Also, the schedule of events must be closely followed, and necessary adjustments must be made in the time frame that was prepared as part of the plan of action.

Just as the careful implementation of the program is essential, so is the monitoring of this phase. Distribution channels must be monitored closely to determine that the program is moving to the market target and is available for exchange. This distribution monitoring is especially important and difficult in health programs that often must depend upon intermediary organizations. Sometimes these groups wish to control communication and materials dissemination from their national headquarters down through their organizational structure to the local chapters. Although this control must be respected, it makes direct monitoring harder and sometimes impossible. More indirect methods, such as observing the flow of the program from local chapters into the community and to the consumer or professional audience, may be hampered by lack of resources to spot-check in the numerous communities that may be involved.

In distributing smoking kits to area physicians for patient counseling, the *County Health Improvement Program* employed two simple, indirect methods of monitoring. A count of total kits that were reported to have been distributed and the number of kits returned by the intermediary organization were compared to the number of physicians in the target area. Secondly, a spot-check of physicians' offices was made to determine how many recalled having received the kits. Based on these measures, it appeared that a number of area physicians had not been covered, and remedial action was begun.

Retail monitoring may also be called for in some health programs. In a pilot test of a program to influence food purchases in cafeterias, the National Heart, Lung, and Blood Institute continuously tracked the cards that were redeemed as part of the incentive game that was employed as well as different information items that were displayed for each food entrée. Other retail areas to be monitored may include prices, point-of-purchase or point-of-decision displays, shelf space, inventory, and competitive reaction. Competition may take many forms. For example, workplace health programs are being offered to corporations in record numbers. Although the commercial and nonprofit offerers of such programs may be concerned with improved employee health and lower health costs, they are competing with each other just as vigorously as two manufacturers fighting over a more traditional market.

The monitoring of sales is another measure of the implementation phase. This includes initial "sell-in," such as the number of hospitals that purchase an audiovisual program or the number of Haitian pharmacies that agree to stock condoms during a program introductory period. Revenues may be part of the sales measure if a program or product is part of a monetary exchange. Also, share-of-market can be part of the sales monitoring process. Goodwill Industries of America, for instance, may wish to know what share of the market it has in a particular city in the training and placement of disabled individuals in local jobs.

Finally, communication must be monitored as part of the process of tracking progress in the marketplace. This may involve verifying the placement of paid and/or public service advertising, quantifying the amount of print and broadcast publicity that was generated, and tracking interpersonal communication. This last element might include the number of presentations made by members of a speakers' bureau, number of village demonstrations held (e.g., for nutrition education in a developing nation), town meetings, school assemblies, and presentations to municipal authorities.

There is another aspect of the implementation phase that requires monitoring. This is the institutional performance of the marketing organization itself. This was a important initial subject of analysis in the first stage of the marketing process. Now it must be monitored to assure that the organization is functioning effectively. This

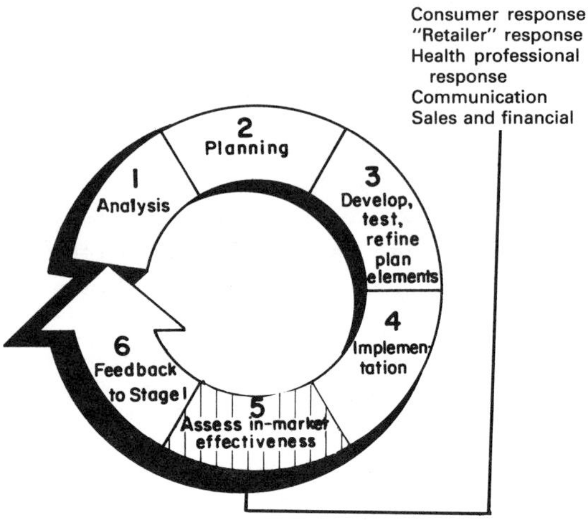

Figure 6. Stage 5 of the marketing process: assessment of in-market effectiveness.

includes staff performance, management attention and response to recommendations, funding, the flow of communication, and the process of decision making. This institutional performance and its monitoring is important in any marketing organization under any circumstances. It is especially critical, however, in health institutions and agencies that are not accustomed to marketing. As discussed elsewhere in this book, health organizations usually are not structured or managed to facilitate marketing decision making. Such circumstances as negative feedback from donors, legislators or other important public figures, reassessment of funding obligations, or a lack of understanding about the continuity that marketing requires can sidetrack a program that otherwise would be successful in the marketplace.

THE FIFTH STAGE—MARKET EFFECTIVENESS

As the implementation proceeds, a systematic assessment is applied to determine the degree to which the marketing program is meeting its objectives; midcourse corrections in the program that may be required to address deficiencies or capitalize on new opportunities, and the extent to which the next cycle of the marketing process must be replanned. The ongoing monitoring in Stage 4 and the continuous assessments in this stage should fit together into an effective management information system.

The purpose of this system is to gather, process, and report timely, adequate, and accurate data for marketing decision making. Part of this system includes a comprehensive internal process for storing and retrieving relevant program information and a marketing intelligence network using members of the distribution force, fieldworkers, or others to gather and send in useful data. Syndicated services and other sources of information may also be tapped, depending upon the nature of the health program and the budget.

On a smaller scale, feedback may be more informal and limited. For instance, the American College of Obstetricians and Gynecologists (ACOG) has developed a self-administered questionnaire that physicians can use to gather information on satisfactions and dissatisfactions from patients. A gynecologist who implements a new service or revises some aspect of his or her practice might utilize the ACOG survey at several points in time to gather and interpret data on patient response.

The program areas in which assessment is needed usually include consumer (i.e., target audience) reaction and response; retailer (or other point of exchange) response; physicians' and other health professionals' responses; communication penetration and impact; and sales and financial measures.

These assessments must be tailored to the individual health program and its objectives. As examples of assessments that may be revised and applied to other health areas, consider the following assessments of in-market effectiveness recommended for contraceptive marketing programs in developing countries:

1. *Consumer response.* Measure and track over time consumer trial of the products, contraceptive buying patterns, user status (i.e., nonuser, potential user, occasional user, regular user, ex-user), usage rate, loyalty status (brand, method), readiness state (unaware, aware, knowledgeable, interested, ready to buy), and satisfactions/dissatisfactions (by product, by consumer segment, by geographic sector/region).
2. *Retailer response.* Establish retail audits and panels to track location of prod-

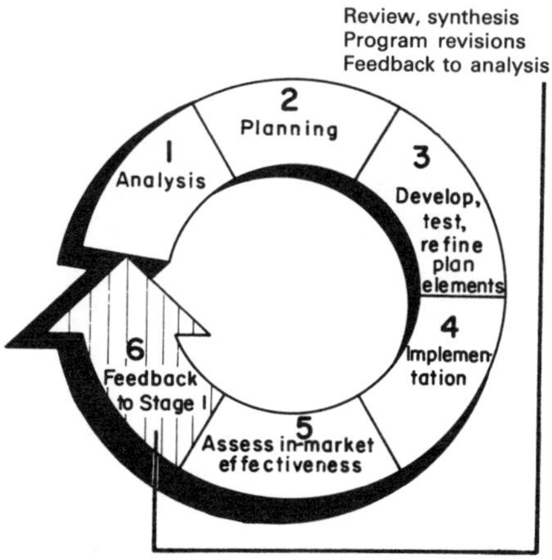

Figure 7. Stage 6 of the marketing process: feedback to Stage 1.

ucts in store (e.g., on shelf, behind counter), reorder rates, trade reaction to incentives, inventories (by product), trade reaction to consumer purchasing behavior, and role of retailers in screening and counseling consumers.

3. *Physicians' and other health professionals' responses.* Measure and track over time reorder rates (of IUDs), number of patient visits for reproductive-related needs, reaction to consumer behavior, and role and reported activities in screening and counseling patients.
4. *Communication.* Use tracking studies to measure periodically awareness, recognition, comprehension, recall, reaction, and perceptions by brand and for overall contraceptive communication.
5. *Sales and financial.* Collect and analyze data in terms of sales, market share, sales-to-expense ratios, and profitability by product, sales territory or other geographic unit, consumer segment, trade channel, and size of order.

THE SIXTH STAGE—FEEDBACK TO STAGE 1

As stated previously, the marketing process is iterative. There can be no let up. The marketplace changes, programs enter phases of decline, and the marketing organization is usually in a state of change as well. The last stage, Stage 6, therefore must feed back into the first.

The monitoring and assessment that occurred in previous stages was undertaken to measure progress, to make program adjustments as needed, and to prepare for replanning. Now, in Stage 6, preparations for this replanning are undertaken. All the information that has been collected includes research, analysis, field intelligence, and other relevant data. This information should be reviewed carefully to uncover problems, identify weaknesses that must be addressed, and identify opportunities that can be exploited in the next cycle.

On the basis of these synthesized data, additional revisions may be undertaken in the marketing program. This procedure of tinkering with the program and making midcourse corrections is a never-ending process that can be undertaken at any point in which it seems necessary at any stage of program development. Finally, all the reviewed data are recycled into Stage 1 (analysis) to begin again the continuous and systematic process of refinement and improvement.

SUMMARY

Marketing, as a framework for achieving organizational objectives by meeting consumer needs and wants, represents a systematic, orderly process for problem solving. This orderly process is well accepted among commercial organizations and has become an almost universal discipline in the private sector. Despite problems with organizational structure, research and analysis, market segmentation, and product and pricing strategies, the same systematic process can be applied to health behavior change.

The marketing process is circular, with the last stage feeding back into the first. Marketing research, the systematic gathering and analysis of information for decision making, is integrated into each stage. The six stages of this marketing process are analysis, planning, development, testing and refining of the plan elements, implementation, assessment of in-market effectiveness, and feedback to Stage 1. These stages incorporate the basic marketing functions of analysis, planning, implementation, and control as well as the marketing actions required to inform, motivate, and service the target markets.

The process is designed to take into account consumer wants, needs, expectations, and satisfactions/dissatisfactions; formulate program objectives; utilize an integrated marketing approach and marketing mix (product, price, communication, distribution); and continuously track consumer and market response.

REFERENCES

Fine, S. *The marketing of ideas and social issues.* New York: Praeger, 1981.

Fox, K. Time as a component of price in social marketing. In *1980 educators' conference proceedings* (Series No. 46). Chicago: American Marketing Association, 1980.

Kotler, P. *Marketing for nonprofit organizations (2nd ed.).* Englewood Cliffs, N.J.: Prentice-Hall, 1982.

National Cancer Institute. *Pretesting in health communications.* (NIH Publication No. 83-1493, Revised December 1982). Washington, D.C.: U.S. Government Printing Office, 1982.

II
Applications

5

The National High Blood Pressure Education Program

An Example of Social Marketing in Action

GRAHAM W. WARD

THE PROBLEM

Hypertension is one of the most prevalent chronic disease conditions in the United States. Approximately 35 million Americans, about 1 in 6, have high blood pressure that warrants some form of treatment. An additional 25 million are estimated to have borderline high blood pressure that requires medical surveillance. Untreated hypertension is the largest single contributor to stroke and a major contributor to heart disease and kidney failure. It is these complications caused by hypertension rather than hypertension itself that generally results in hospitalization. Hypertension is more common among blacks than whites—about 1 out of 4 blacks has definite high blood pressure, contrasted to 1 in 6 in the general population.

In addition to being a major accelerating factor in the 500,000 strokes (175,000 stroke deaths) and 1,250,000 heart attacks (650,000 heart attack deaths) each year, hypertensive heart disease, hypertension, and ischemic heart disease with hypertension accounted for more than 90,000 deaths in the U.S. in 1976. Although

GRAHAM W. WARD • School of Medicine, Tufts University, Boston, Massachusetts 02111.

direct hypertension deaths are a gross underestimate of the effect of hypertension on overall cardiovascular disease mortality, they clearly indicate its significance.

Actuarial, epidemiologic, and clinical data confirm that the risk of subsequent illness and/or death increases with blood pressure. Even within the normal blood pressure ranges the relationship persists: A person with a blood pressure of 130/80 is at greater risk of premature death or illness from heart failure, heart attack, stroke, and kidney failure than an individual with a blood pressure of 110/70. These risks begin to accelerate at about a level of 140/90, a level now accepted as the arbitrary threshold of borderline hypertension.

The specific causes of 90% to 95% of hypertension remain unknown. We do not yet know enough about the fundamental processes involved to prevent or cure it. Thus, short-term emphasis must be placed on optimizing control of existing hypertension. Studies indicate that lowering blood pressure with drugs is possible on a long-term basis and that this results in less illness and fewer deaths. In some individuals, nutritional changes such as salt and weight control may lessen the degree of or even obviate the need for drug therapy.

In 1972, the nation faced a contradictory situation vis-à-vis hypertension control. On the one hand, therapies effective in lowering blood pressure and its dreadful complications were available. On the other hand, within the large population of hypertensive patients, many were not aware of their condition, some were receiving treatment, but only a few were successfully controlling their blood pressure.

There were many reasons for the failure to control hypertension. For example, the public and professionals alike tended to minimize the serious nature of all but severe hypertension. The health hazard represented by even mild hypertension was not clearly recognized. Among professionals, confusion existed in selecting among a multitude of drugs, each with a differing mode of action. Additionally, most professional publications on hypertension focused on the diagnosis of the few cases of secondary hypertension and neglected the management of essential hypertension—the ultimate diagnosis in more than 90% of our nation's 35 million hypertensive patients. Finally, regimen adherence issues were poorly addressed by both physicians and patients.

In summary, hypertension has been recognized as a serious chronic disease condition of massive proportions. Effective treatment procedures have been demonstrated to be effective in controlling high blood pressure. The problem thus became defined in terms of community education. How could effective treatment strategies for hypertension be transmitted to professionals and the public? The specific goals included (1) increasing public awareness of the problem of hypertension and (2) motivating diagnosed hypertensives to comply with medication regimens and other behavioral strategies for reducing and maintaining blood pressure at acceptable levels. To achieve these two interrelated goals, the National Heart, Lung, and Blood Institute launched a large-scale multidisciplinary program named the *National High Blood Pressure Education Program* (NHBPEP) in 1972.

MARKET ANALYSIS

It would be nice to say that a full detailed marketing analysis program existed in 1972 so that a textbook case could be presented here. This was not the case; there were no applicable textbooks at that time. We did some homework nonetheless, some of it in the early stages, but much of it in later bits and pieces as the program staff developed insights and gleaned resources to implement those insights.

The fielding of a national baseline survey of public knowledge, attitudes, and reported behaviors vis-à-vis high blood pressure was an early major step taken in 1973. This survey (replicated in 1979 for evaluation purposes) confirmed some suspicions, neatly popped the balloons of some conventional wisdom, and brought to light some problems that had not been anticipated. To highlight these quickly:

1. *Suspicions confirmed*—Hypertension was seen as only a moderately serious condition; hypertension as a cause of illness was well perceived, but its control was not identified as a preventive measure; the public used a large array of sources for health information, leaning most heavily on health professionals and then on the electronic media.
2. *Conventional wisdom deflated*—Screening as a major need was sharply contradicted by the finding that over 75% of the sample had had a blood pressure check within 12 months; cost of medication, a strongly decried barrier to following therapy, was found to be a minor factor for most persons.
3. *Some surprises*—Many therapy dropouts said their physician told them to stop; the magnitude of confusion between hypertension and nervous tension was far greater than expected; many people appeared to use false cues (e.g., tension) as a guide to taking medication.

Health professionals (although physicians were later surveyed directly) were approached differently. Four task forces were created in 1972 for the purpose of developing a consensus on a definition of hypertension and its therapy, professional education needs, community education needs, and a resources impact assessment. (This latter point was due to concern over what would happen if all the then-estimated 23 million hypertensives came out of the woodwork. The 1973 survey described previously later showed that many were already out.) Although constituted ostensibly as planning groups, these task forces served in many ways like the focus groups often used by marketers to test concepts. The consensus on proposed actions that emerged represented quite directly what was acceptable to a variety of health professionals and/or their organizations, what products they wished to see developed, what price (usually in convenience cost terms) they would be willing to pay for those products, and how they wished the products to be delivered.

Data were also gathered on patient visits for hypertension (and for all causes) and for antihypertensive prescribing rates. At the time, no one knew whether these numbers should or could change rapidly, slowly, or at all, but it was clear that some measure of motion in the market was required. These measures proved appropriate, and they have now been followed for a decade as one guide to program decision making.

This early adopted fact gathering and consensus process has been continued as an ongoing effort throughout the program's life. Additional large- and small-scale surveys of the public were taken several times. A survey of physicians was mounted in 1977. There has been continuous monitoring of data on deaths, patient visits, and prescribing patterns. A variety of data from the National Center for Health Statistics, especially the Health Interview Surveys and the Health and Nutrition Examination Surveys, have been drawn upon heavily. Dozens of professional consensus groups have been sponsored. A materials pretesting system and use of consumer focus groups were both adopted as routine action about 1975–1976. A full detailing of all data gathered and the findings in those data would fill far more than this marketing text.

DEVELOPING THE PROGRAM

The existing health care system contains inadequate mechanisms both for accomplishing and for financing detection and treatment of high blood pressure for large segments of the population. Existing means for continuing education of health professionals are often poorly organized and rarely relate to a demonstrated educational need. Lacking at times are resources and mechanisms to accomplish long-term (chronic) patient education and follow-up or any significant amount of consumer education. A large and sometimes disproportionate reliance must be placed on voluntary activity to accomplish these tasks. This often leads to extreme variance in quality and considerable discontinuity of effort. Thus, a well-coordinated interdisciplinary effort was viewed as holding the greatest promise for meeting the challenge posed by the serious problem of hypertension.

The NHBPEP, although coordinated by the National Heart, Lung, and Blood Institute (NHLBI) of the National Institutes of Health (NIH), is not a single-agency activity. Rather, it is an ever-growing coalition of some 15 federal agencies, 150 national professional, voluntary, and trade organizations, nearly all state and many local public health departments, and over 2,000 organized community programs. Insurance companies, pharmaceutical firms, and many other private industries play increasingly active roles in this program as do many organized labor organizations. Nor can one omit countless numbers of individual physicians, nurses, pharmacists, health educators, and other health professionals in whose private offices most hypertensive patients are detected, treated, and counseled. Hundreds of television stations, thousands of radio stations, newspapers, and magazines have been important to the overall effort by carrying the hypertension control message to the nation.

When first organized, the *National High Blood Pressure Education Program* concentrated on two activities that can be well described in marketing terms. Data available at that time suggested that about half the people then defined as having hypertension did not know it—in spite of the fact that over three quarters of the population reported blood pressure checks within the year. If physicians told their clients about blood pressure, the message was not retained. Many of those aware of their high blood pressure were not being treated, and many of those being treated did not have their high blood pressure controlled, thus suggesting lack of attention by both client and providers (Ward, 1976). Awareness, therefore, was a prime concern. In marketing terms, we had a *promotion* problem. We had to make high blood pressure interesting or at least noticeable.

A second activity dealt with the task of establishing a network of interested organizations and individuals through whom we could distribute information to health professionals and their clients. Expressed as one of the four *p*'s, it was a *place* problem. Our program's product—hypertension control information and technology—had to have local outlets to assure its accessibility in the community. Place, in the marketing problem we were attempting to solve, did not turn out to be a simple, discrete entity related only to distribution. Rather, it was highly interwoven with the concept of *price*. Convenience costs rather than monetary costs (i.e., easy access to services or information rather than the price of a prescription or office visit) seemed more a barrier to action. In some communities, this problem was more readily solved by simple promotion of more convenient services that already existed but were not widely known. In most instances, it was necessary to foster community-based planning efforts to modify old or to create new services. The astute marketer will quickly recognize that selling community-based planning for hypertension control generates its own set of marketing strategy needs. Those details, however, exceed the overview intended in this chapter.

The marketing concept of *product* creates a challenging, twofold problem for such programs as the *National High Blood Pressure Education Program*. First, the primary products, as seen in the community, are a variety of health care and health counseling services that are neither produced nor delivered by the NHBPEP. Nevertheless, we want to influence their quality and distribution. Secondly, these service products must be distinguished from the education materials and consultation products produced under the control of the program staff but usually delivered by others.

Product, like place, is also interwoven with price in several respects. A consensus-developed educational product (e.g., the Report of the Joint National Committee on Detection, Evaluation and Treatment of High Blood Pressure, 1977) that bore the endorsement of key physician groups participating in the consensus helped reduce the price (hazard of violating peer group norms) and contributed to greater and more rapid physician adoption of the recommendations.

A second impact of product on perceived price arises from well-considered development, preferably including pretesting, of educational materials that makes products easier for the consumer to use. This is especially true for the busy health care provider. Physicians, pharmacists, nurses, and others have minimal free time to stay up to date in their fields. Thus, the NHBPEP attempted from the beginning to produce concise, logical, and simply written materials that digested the essence of new findings rather than give exhaustive but relatively uninformative bibliographies. The intent of this effort was to reduce the time and energy cost of learning and to enhance the likelihood that recommended changes in practice would be adopted.

For the general public, the cost barrier was dealt with by attempting to increase the perceived costs of inaction, in addition to seeking real reductions in convenience costs. We used high fear arousal initially, then shifted to more positive presentations. Thus, a constant element of publically directed messages has been cataloging the often catastrophic results of *not* controlling high blood pressure, namely, heart disease, strokes, and kidney disease. Positioned against this are painless detection of the problem and simple, daily therapies that control blood pressure with minimal interference with normal activities. In short, we could not lower the monetary price of treatment, but we could and did try to increase the perceived value for what was bought at that price.

Segmenting the Market

Market segmentation is probably the most complex question of all marketing factors for the NHBPEP. It starts simply enough by stating that the program is trying to reach, relatively simultaneously, three broad groups: health care providers who manage hypertensive patients, persons who have hypertension, and the general public.

Providers must be further segmented by profession, type of facility or practice in which they work, and geographic region. They may have to be segmented by age or ethnic group on occasion. To take advantage of existing dissemination channels, it is often necessary to segment providers by professional society affiliation.

Patients, or more specifically, persons having high blood pressure are initially segmented into two groups: those aware that they have hypertension and those who are not yet aware. The former group is further divided into those remaining in treatment who must be reinforced to stay there; those formerly in treatment who must be persuaded to resume therapy; and those who never began treatment who must be persuaded to do so.

Even the vast general public cannot be considered monolithic. We must divide this massive group. Some individuals will know or be related to people having hypertension; these must be taught how to provide supportive encouragement to help people with hypertension to enter, reenter, or continue treatment. Some may, at a later time, acquire hypertension and must be prepared to deal with it rationally. Some may wish to take action, to the extent it is possible, to avoid acquiring high blood pressure. Both patients and the general public are further segmented by age, sex, ethnic group, education, and whether they live in rural or metropolitan areas.

For all these professional, patient, and public segments, hypertension has a different significance and represents a different problem to be solved. The actions each group must take and the skills required to perform those actions are different. The mix of channels and the execution of the message to reach each group are different and must be taken into account if we are to transmit most effectively the problem, the solution, and the skills required to implement the solution.

This already complex mix of audiences is made more complicated because the NHBPEP cannot reach them all directly. Communicating with hundreds of millions of the public, tens of millions of patients, and hundreds of thousands of providers requires the use of intermediaries. The NHBPEP goal, in fact, is to establish the role of these intermediaries so well that the NHLBI can eventually relinquish much of its present leadership role in hypertension control education. Although the initial role of the intermediary groups is to serve as a communications channel, identifying and recruiting the assistance of these groups required a similar market analysis and segmentation. The full listing is too lengthy to present here, but types of groups include professional societies, voluntary health organizations, civic and service groups, organized labor and management organizations, state and local health departments, drug, insurance, and other private corporations, other federal agencies, and over 2,000 locally organized hypertension control programs.

PROGRAM DESCRIPTION

High Blood Pressure Information Center

A key focal point within the program and the program's primary interface with the general public and health professionals is the High Blood Pressure Information Center. The center answers public inquiries about high blood pressure and distributes free educational materials, short reports, bibliographies and studies, posters, radio and television materials, reprints, and other items. The information center also acts as a clearinghouse for similar materials prepared by nongovernment sources, for relevant articles in the professional literature, and for community and state programmatic activities. It schedules educational exhibits for both professional and lay group meetings and conventions. A speaker's roster provides lecturers who are knowledgeable about high blood pressure or helps organizations find qualified speakers in their own localities. The center annually receives approximately 125,000 individual inquiries and distributes well over 1 million pieces of informational material.

Community Program Development

On request, the Community Program Development Service offers technical assistance to help community organizations to develop plans for improved efforts to control high blood pressure. The service draws on federal government experts and on experienced practitioners from successful community programs. Periodically, the service sponsors special invitational workshops; it also helps communities to develop their own workshops. For the past several years, activities of this component have been managed and coordinated using states as working units primarily because institute resources available to the program are inadequate to reach all community programs on an individual basis. Some 2,000 active community programs have been identified.

Educational Materials Assessment

The program reviews and endorses, on request, public and professional educational materials developed by any source. The program logo and the phrase "prepared in cooperation with the *National High Blood Pressure Education Program*" can be included on these materials if they meet these criteria: The items must not be sold for profit, must contain no product endorsement, and must be technically accurate.

Professional Education

Recommendations for detection, treatment, and patient education have been developed for the program by nationally recognized experts. These recommendations are the basis for both content of a variety of professional education materials developed by the program and for those developed by many other sources. This activity relates closely to and maintains liaison with a variety of groups, including major professional organizations such as the American and National Medical associations, American and National Dental associations, American and National Nurses associations, American and National Pharmaceutical associations, American Association of Medical Colleges, National Board of Medical Examiners, American Academy of Family Physicians, American College of Cardiology, American Heart Association, and pharmaceutical companies.

Public Education

The program coordinates a cooperative public education effort involving both local and national organizations and the media. The primary function of this component is to develop and coordinate distribution of mass media materials. In past years, the institute has acquired $3 to $5 million annually in free public service advertising space. When the success of other participating groups is added to this figure, it is not unreasonable to estimate that as much as $20 million worth of free public service announcement (PSA) space and time on radio and television and in print materials is garnered each year. This estimate does not include value impact of booklets, leaflets, flyers, and posters distributed by the institute's High Blood Pressure Information Center and the many other participant organizations each year.

Patient Education

The program has taken the posture that patient education is a requisite component of therapy and that control of high blood pressure eventually evolves to an irreducible two-member team of patient and provider. The concept that the patient is a member of the health care team is considered vital. Many organizations participating within the program have developed and distributed patient education materials. The institute has been involved in developing effective methods for pretesting these materials prior to their distribution. In addition, the institute and several other participating groups are actively involved in motivating health care providers to engage actively and effectively in patient education activities. As an example, institute-supported curriculum and materials development have been provided, in collaboration with the American Academy of Family Practitioners and the Society of Teachers of Family Medicine, to assist improved training of family practice residents in patient education.

Minority Populations

The program has long recognized the unique needs of the variety of minority populations in the United States. In 1975, the program held its first National Forum on Hypertension Among Minority Communities, and it conducted a second national forum in 1980. An outcome of the first forum was establishment of an ongoing Ad Hoc Committee on Hypertension in Minority Populations that has directed workshops for many minority groups, including Native Americans, Asian Americans, blacks, and Hispanic-origin groups including Puerto Ricans, Cubans, and Mexican Americans. In addition, for 2 years the institute supported a Black Health Providers Task Force whose recommendations presented at a White House conference may have considerable impact on the delivery of hypertension care services to black populations.

School Health Education

School health education is a new effort that will be developed during the coming years. A multitude of studies have shown that the adult population is frequently ill informed about the health care system, the functions of the body, and the nature of health risk factors. Although lifelong reinforcement of health messages can never be eliminated, this activity can be substantially reduced if all children learn in their basic primary and secondary schools both the current essentials of these topics and how to interpret and apply new health information as it is developed. The function of this program area is not to engage directly in school health education activities but rather to work with persons in the field of education toward improving health curricula and positioning the NHLBI and other organizations participating in the program as resources for school health education.

Educational Research Grants Program

The scientific base for developing effective educational programs for the public, patients, and health professionals is still developing. A major interest of the program is the conduct of educational research and the exploration of innovative, cost-effective ways of using education as a primary tool to gain greater control of high blood pressure. The institute has, since 1974, provided continuing support to a variety of grants performing such research.

Demonstration Projects

The NHLBI has developed three major demonstration areas. These are (1) statewide coordination of high blood pressure control; (2) high blood pressure control at the work setting; and (3) community high blood pressure control demonstration projects. The statewide projects are intended to assess the impact of resource/activity coordination upon the hypertension control status of patients and upon selected morbidity and mortality outcomes. Workplace demonstrations will assist the ability of industry to mount and evaluate programs to detect hypertension, educate employees, and maintain hypertension control, as well as to ascertain costs of such efforts. An additional project explored the role of health insurers in stimulating and assisting development of worksite-based hypertension education and control programs. The Community Demonstration Program is examining models for implementation at the local level and is measuring outcomes of both health care status and operational costs. Model sites have been chosen in both urban and rural areas.

Special Studies and Evaluation

To provide baseline evaluation data and to acquire planning information, the institute has supported a variety of special studies of varying scope and depth and has made an active effort to secure data from other sources for this purpose. Examples of major studies supported include two national samples of the general public (1973 and 1979) to determine existing knowledge, attitudes, and behavior related to high blood pressure. Under the auspices of the Food and Drug Administration, a similar study was conducted among physicians in 1978. Other studies include examination of the relationship between high blood pressure and life insurance, characteristics of automated blood pressure measuring devices, employment policies related to high blood pressure, and state health department high blood pressure activities. A key study concerns the cost/benefits of high blood pressure therapy; it is contemplated that this study will be revised and refined on a continuing basis as a tool for assisting national and community program planning.

PROGRAM RESULTS AND IMPLICATIONS

Since the inception of the *National High Blood Pressure Education Program,* few would deny that there has been substantial, measurable progress in hypertension control in the United States. This progress has been achieved only by the willing participation of many individuals and organizations, a willingness derived from presentation of convincing arguments based on sound data that (1) a real problem exists; (2) practical solutions exist; (3) benefits are likely if the solutions are implemented; and (4) progress was made that was commensurate with the implementation investment.

We have not yet won the war, but we have pushed the front forward a long way. There are many indicators of progress. The NHLBI conducted comparison surveys for the years 1973 and 1979 to find out how much the public had learned about high blood pressure and its treatment and what it was doing with that knowledge (Haines & Ward, 1981). The comparison of 1979 to 1973 surveys showed the following:

- Sixteen percent more people know that hypertension is a very serious disease.
- Thirty-three percent more people have come to understand that high blood pressure and hypertension mean the same thing.
- Nineteen percent more people know that hypertension can cause strokes.

- Sixty-six percent more people know that normal blood pressure is less than 140/90.
- Twenty-seven percent fewer hypertensive persons had trouble getting life insurance.
- Forty-three percent fewer hypertensives missed work due to high blood pressure.
- Eighty-three percent (1979) versus 78% (1973) of the public had its blood pressure checked within a year.
- Eighty-two percent (1979) versus 77% (1973) of hypertensives still take the medication prescribed for them.

A key indicator that has increased appreciably is patient visits for hypertension. Visits for hypertension rose 10% from 1972 to 1980, whereas visits for all causes actually fell 13% during the same period (Ward, 1981). The proportion of persons who have hypertension and know they have this usually symptomless condition rose from 51% in 1971–1972 immediately before the *National High Blood Pressure Education Program* was inaugurated to 68% in 1974–1975, the last year for which national data are available. This is progress, but it leaves 32% of those with high blood pressure who still must be found. At the same time, what is perhaps the most difficult task—achieving long-term control—has begun to show substantial movement upward, from 16.5% under control in 1971–1972 to 24.2% in 1974–1975 (Ward, 1981).

The real payoff and goal of the NHBPEP is the reduction of illness, disability, and death from high blood pressure. Specifics on changes each year in the number of heart attacks, strokes, and other complications of high blood pressure would be helpful, but such information simply does not exist. A onetime study by the National Institute of Neurological and Communicative Disorders and Stroke has suggested that the standardized incidence ratio of first strokes declined about 15% from 1971 to 1976. It appears that there is some basis for optimism in that regard (Ward, 1981).

Information on mortality rates *is* available and is highly encouraging. The cause of death most closely associated with hypertension is stroke. The age-adjusted stroke death rate has been dropping for decades—about 1% each year in the 1950s and 1½% to 2% each year during the 1960s. Since the effort to increase hypertension control began in 1972, this decline has grown to over 5% each year and continues to fall. In other words, the age-adjusted stroke death rate fell 30% from 1972 to 1978 (Levy & Ward, 1979).

Although the temporal relationship is strong, one cannot accurately determine how much hypertension control has contributed to this decline. Our citizens also smoke less, have changed their eating habits, are more physically active, and receive better medical care. All these factors doubtless contribute as well. But scientists at the NHLBI and many of their research and clinical colleagues, knowing too well the ravages of uncontrolled hypertension, believe that its improved control has played a significant role in this change (Levy & Ward, 1979).

The decade of experience in persuading the nation to take action on hypertension control has yielded some general principles that are applicable to many if not most prevention efforts.

Strong Science Base

The ultimate success of any prevention effort can be no greater than the effectiveness of the intervention used. With only a few exceptions, most of the technologies or approaches used to prevent disease must be used by a very large proportion of individual citizens. Promotion of such widescale application, irrespective of how small the unit cost may be, requires a relatively high degree of certainty that the approach does provide a benefit commensurate with its cost and with its risk. Assessing these attributes usually requires an in-depth understanding of the abnormal disease process. This, in turn, requires an understanding of normal body processes.

Hypertension represents an excellent example of this issue. Although scientists have gained enough understanding to control this condition and to prevent its complications in large measure, they cannot now prevent or cure hypertension itself because they do not know its cause or causes. Such primary prevention, rather than the secondary prevention offered by control, is the ultimate goal.

Program Data Base

Before the program could move effectively to increase hypertension control through public and professional education, it had to ascertain how many people had hypertension, knew they had it, were being treated actively, and were well controlled. It had to assess knowledge levels of the public, patients, and their care providers. It had to determine what organizations and agencies were already pursuing hypertension control and what they were doing. It had to learn what sources all these people turned to when they wanted the kind of information the program had to give them. Thus, in addition to scientific knowledge and before engaging in any educational or marketing activity, either major and sweeping or detailed with limited scope, a critical mass of operational information had to be obtained. For this and for any similar effort, sufficient, clear data must be obtained to allow identification of problems and subproblems to permit the setting of concrete objectives and to allow the problem and its nature and extent to be shared with and understood by many individuals. It is necessary to gain knowledge about the range of intervention options that are available and the extent to which these options have been tested and proved beneficial. Equally essential is the identification of persons within organizations or as individuals who are in a position to effect the interventions, the specific roles they must play, and the skills they must have to play these roles. Redundant communication channels to reach these various actors must be identified so that they may be made aware of the problem and their potential roles in its solution. A further reason for explicitly defining a problem and its components is the need to develop measurable indicators of progress. It is impossible to track progress in solving any problem if one does not understand its starting status well.

Realistic Time Frame and Expectations

Another lesson learned in the operation of the *National High Blood Pressure Education Program* is the value of seeking progress in small increments. Hypertension control requires that four broad functions are completed: (1) detecting the person who has high blood pressure, (2) bringing that individual under active care, (3) selecting the best treatment for that individual, and (4) maintaining that therapy, usually for life. The program has been unable to move the nation to address each of these steps simultaneously with equal vigor. That is why more people are detected (aware of their condition) than are controlled.

As a general concept, major social problems are usually not subject to revolutionary change. Rather, to maintain stability within a system and to achieve accepted change that is lasting, an evolutionary, incremental process must be established. A precondition to success of the evolution is a commitment to sustain the effort for the required period of time and to engender among program operators and program service recipients a high degree of patience, which is tempered by realistic expectations of the achievable rate of change. Had the *National High Blood Pressure Education Program* been forced to demonstrate a major impact after the first, second, or even third year of operation as a basis for its continued survival, the program would not be alive today.

An absolute requirement in selecting specific goals and directions for a program is to recognize that some probable absolute limits of accomplishment exist. If goals and objectives are to be realistic, they must be based on realistic expectations of what can be accomplished within an existing state of the art and within practical limits on the quantity and quality of resources that can be made available.

A simplistic analysis illustrates the need for such a perspective. Under most circumstances, hypertension control can be described as the accomplishment of four basic and sequential steps. These are (1) detection (the recognition of an elevated blood pressure suggesting the presence of hypertension), (2) referral (a term intended here to mean the several actions necessary to achieve definitive diagnosis and to bring a patient under active medical care), (3) selection of appropriate therapy, and (4) long-term maintenance of that therapy and blood pressure control. To control hyper-

Table 1. High Blood Pressure Control Process: Alternative Probabilities

	Event probability	Overall probability
Detection	.85	.85
Referral	.85	.72
Correct therapy	.85	.61
Maintain control (2 years)	.85	.52

tension successfully in a given patient, each of these steps must be accomplished in the sequence presented. Each step has a probability of being accomplished. Or, stated somewhat differently, each step will be completed successfully only in a certain percentage of occasions. The net effectiveness of the hypertension control process can be expressed as the product of the probabilities of each step. If one assumes a high but less-than-perfect rate of accomplishment of each step, let us say a probability of .85 for each, then the probability of completing all steps is only .52 (see Table 1).

The implication of this simple analysis is that, achieving each step with 85% efficiency—probably the highest reasonably expectable rate without reaching diminishing returns on economic investment—it may not be realistic to expect to have under control at any given point in time more than about half of the true hypertensive population. Only by eliminating one of the steps, possibly by combining detection and referral, can one eliminate a multiplier and thereby significantly increase the yield of the effort. Even then, expectations must be limited. Such a three-step process with a probability of .85 accomplishment of each step yields a total product of approximately .61 or 61% effectiveness. This analysis is intended to be illustrative, not definitive. Nonetheless, it indicates that projections of outcome goals and objectives must be done cautiously and conservatively.

Leveraging Resources

It was clear from the beginning of the effort that the NHLBI would never have sufficient resources to solve, singlehandedly, the problems in hypertension control that had to be met. From the first day of the NHBPEP, the program worked to recruit the resources of other parties, to use our dollars to move the greater amount of dollars others had. For the practice the program uses the financial term *leveraging*.

Leveraging can take many forms. Persons familiar with research, particularly operations research, will know of the Hawthorne effect. According to the Hawthorne effect, just letting people know someone is interested and watching can influence a situation. Making federal interest in hypertension control widely known, thereby legitimizing the issue by lending it credibility, is an important factor in achieving the changes associated with the NHBPEP. Although support for action is undoubtedly important, massive outlay of federal dollars is not always the most effective way to bring about some changes. An example of this is the response to the Report of the Joint National Committee on Detection, Evaluation, and Treatment of High Blood Pressure. The support cost for producing and distributing this committee report was miniscule in terms of typical federal outlays. Yet, the interest and change generated by the output of this committee has likely been greater than a multimillion dollar aid program.

A second leveraging approach is use of the consensus process. If a wide variety of persons or organizations must make a similar response to a similar problem, inviting active participation of those organizations to define the problem and recommend the response greatly increases the likelihood that the organizations will perform as desired. Such developmental participation also tends to make the organizations advocates of the recommendations and expands the cadre of communicators and persuaders on the issue. Consensus also has some disadvantages. It is a slow process. It also usually requires compromise among those involved. Thus, the result is only rarely the best. Rather, it is as good as is possible at the time. Reiterations of the process over time must be done to approach the optimum gradually as people gather new information or become accustomed to new ideas and find them workable. Decisive action comes, but it comes in small increments over time. (Neither coordination nor consensus necessarily means selling the program but rather, our objective is to stimulate interest in and action upon high blood pressure control irrespective of whether individuals or groups choose to ally themselves with the organization now known as the *National High Blood Pressure Education Program.*)

A more typical approach to leveraging often used by the program is persuading other organizations to use their influence or resources to advance the program's cause. This approach is successful only to the extent that the organization being recruited can genuinely profit in some respect by participating. Altruistic motives are usually short-lived and too fickle to be dependable. A clear profit motive (e.g., increased productivity, increased sales, improved visibility in the community or market area) is a much more solid basis for sustained effort. The NHBPEP has been very fortunate in finding partners, such as local governments, voluntary agencies, professional societies, labor unions, and a host of commercial enterprises, who could perceive such a payoff. Indeed, a good 90% of the resources now being applied to hypertension control come from these partners, not the federal government.

Source Credibility

Another major lesson learned by the staff members of the program is the importance of source credibility. Thus far, most persons would agree that the NHBPEP enjoys the reputation of having its facts in order. Although the program does not always move rapidly, it undeniably moves surely. The time invested to complete the homework necessary for thorough problem analysis has consistently proved to be an investment with high payoff.

Minimizing Directives

Closely associated with source credibility is another approach that has long been used by the program and has high receptivity. The approach uses questions rather than answers, to avoid being overly directive and thus resisted. Since the inception of the program, we have experienced an incessant demand for planning models. Because the situation in a given community or organization is so unique in terms of level of interest, resources available, relations among organizations and communities, distribution and availability of health care services, and a variety of other aspects, no single model nor even a series of several alternative models has adequate specificity. Recognizing this inadequacy of models, which are, in effect, proposed solutions or answers to a problem, the program turned early to a mode that employed questions rather than answers. If a community sought assistance in some aspect of hypertension control, program staff attempted to supply a list of key questions that would provide that community with its own unique and specific operational model, if answered from the unique perspective of that community.

It turns out that states and communities are filled with bright, energetic people who strongly resist having an externally made solution to their problems forced upon them. Given a modicum of help to sort their problems into manageable pieces, they frequently develop highly imaginative solutions that could be conceived only by an insider. This approach has been effective in at least two ways: (1) Communities or organizations would not delay exploring hypertension control opportunities because the proffered model did not clearly fit their situation, and (2) the use of questions did not create the appearance that the federal government was telling communities what to do but, rather, was offering useful assistance.

Emphasis on "How To"

A further lesson to be learned is that the NHBPEP is an educational, not an informational, program. This distinction is important. Providing information that a problem exists and describing its parameters is rarely adequate to achieve appropriate action on the part of the many individuals who must act to solve the problem. Insofar as the state of the art permits, the program has made a clear effort to emphasize *teaching skills,* to transmit not only information but capabilities. Although such an effort requires greater time to develop and greater time to market, it must be made. If people understand only what is to be done but not how to do it, the only action one may obtain is the wringing of hands and the issuing of exhortive statements. Only by continuing to teach how-to skills will any program achieve its goals and establish a legacy of ongoing, productive action that is not dependent on government.

Using What We Have

The importance of using the existing health care system rather than attempting to establish a separate and distinct prevention care system cannot be overstated. Efforts to achieve the latter would result only in frustration arising from further fragmentation of care and the development of activities that are unlikely to become self-supporting. Until the entire structure of the health care delivery system in the United States is modified, we must continue to recognize that there is but one health care system and that its primary mode of support is fee for service. Hypertension control or any other preventive care program must be solidly integrated into this system. Any other approach will only create unending demands for extra, massive support that our society cannot provide on the necessary sustained basis.

The Need to Sell

The world does not automatically beat a path to the better mousetrap inventor. Research can sometimes be an expensive process, but nonetheless it is one that brings a severalfold return on investment *if its results are applied.* Scientific knowledge, like any other commodity in our economy, must be marketed if it is to be adopted rapidly and widely. This implies a postresearch investment to make the marketing dissemination happen. The resources required are not large, in contrast to most federal expenditures or to the results achieved. Neither are they inconsequential. For the past 5 years, the NHLBI educational effort in hypertension has cost about $3 million each year. That is equivalent to 5 cents a year for each of the 60 million Americans at risk due to high blood pressure. The NHLBI has begun to taper *that* amount down as more and more private sector resources become permanently invested in high blood pressure control.

It is difficult to establish a formula that automatically specifies the level of needed resources for a prevention effort, nor can one usually predict at the outset the likely mix of public and private investment needed to enhance success. It seems clear, however, that establishing a basic coordinated effort is indispensable.

In the case of the NHBPEP, the core-funding level at the NHLBI was determined primarily by estimating coordination requirements: identification of the sectors in society whose activity was needed and the functions required to link those sectors. Because many elements in our society do not normally interact directly, we believe a legitimate federal role, the role the NHLBI has adopted, is that of a linchpin, brokering information, experiences, and ideas among these disparate elements. More of the program budget is used for this purpose than for direct production of educational materials that can be and are increasingly produced by local government and the private sector. Although the NHLBI dollar investment has not risen substantially over the years, the dollar investment of those in the private sector who have been persuaded to join the overall effort has rapidly multiplied.

SUSTAINING SUCCESS

Sustaining hard-won changes as ongoing, normative modes of action brings some additional concerns into play. As a program matures, it faces more difficult problems that may require additional resources, development of new technology, new organization of health services delivery (which may require new kinds of personnel or new professional relationships to accomplish), and other measures that will contribute to the long-term institutionalization of the remaining required changes.

In addition, a program faces increasing difficulty in sustaining interest after the initial novelty has worn off. In the case of the NHBPEP, the program has matured far beyond the bandwagon stage of development. With increasing frequency, the program staff members must walk a finer and finer line as they seek to make the desired elements of hypertension control commonplace occurrences while avoiding development of a nonchalant attitude before many important tasks are completed. At the same time, participants in the program who have retained their enthusiasm—or at least their doggedness—become discouraged because they believe that an increasing number of people and organizations have come to view hypertension control as passé. In many instances, however, this may be viewed as an indicator of success because new ideas and activities have become accepted as ordinary.

In summary, prevention efforts can succeed in a cost-effective fashion provided that

1. the goals sought have proven value that stand the test of time;
2. the interventions used have proven value;
3. program planning uses data rather than intuition to the extent possible;
4. adequate resources are invested over a realistic period of time;
5. sound marketing principles are used; and
6. the activities and policies of disparate participants are coordinated into a whole and the coordinator has received wide credibility.

SUMMARY

What do we know from our experience with the NHBPEP? We know that a clear public health problem exists and that it impacts a sizable fraction of the population in terms of health and economics. We know that there are at least partial solutions to this problem that require acceptance and action by large numbers of diverse persons. In marketing terms, there are applicable products. The products are not universally sought or used (a promotion problem). The products are not universally available (a place problem). The cost of the products is not usually prohibitive, but the value at whatever cost is not always perceived as high (a price problem).

These factors allow the problem to be addressed in marketing terms and pursued by employing marketing methods. This has been done for the last decade with sizable positive results that have surprised even the marketers. The process works but only when it is diligently followed and when such data as are available are believed and are used in the process. The process works when the market is logically segmented and when the opinions, wants, needs, and inclinations of each segment are identified and incorporated into action strategies. Most importantly, the process works when the problem is clearly identified and when solutions are allowed to emerge from problem analysis rather than from intuition or tradition. Social marketing hath its charm; it can be a lethal charm if misapplied, a balm when done correctly.

REFERENCES

Haines, C., & Ward, G. Recent trends in public knowledge, attitudes and reported behavior with respect to high blood pressure. *Public Health Reports,* 1981, *96*(6), 514–522.

Levy, R., & Ward, G. Hypertension control: A succeeding national effort. *Journal of the American Medical Association,* 1979, *241*(23), 2546.

Report of the Joint National Committee on the Detection, Evaluation, and Treatment of High Blood Pressure: A Cooperative Study. *Journal of the American Medical Association,* 1977, *237,* 255–261.

Ward, G. , Testimony before U.S. Senate Committee on Labor and Human Resources, July 16, 1981.

Ward, G. & Johnson, R. Recent trends in hypertension control. *Urban Health,* 1976, *5*(3), 38–39.

BIBLIOGRAPHY

Prevalence Data

Hypertension in adults 25–74 years of age, United States, 1971–1975 (Vital and Health Statistics, Series II, Number 221, Department of Health and Human Services Publication No. [PHS] 81-1671). Washington, D.C.: U.S. Government Printing Office, 1981.

Mortality Trends

Five-Year Findings of the Hypertension Detection and Follow-up Program. 1. Reduction in Mortality of Persons with High Blood Pressure, Including Mild Hypertension. 2. Mortality by Race-Sex and Age. *Journal of the American Medical Association,* 1979, *242,* 2562–2577.

Proceedings of the conference on the decline in coronary heart disease mortality (USDHEW Publication No. [PHS]

79-1610, National Institutes of Health). Washington, D.C.: U.S. Government Printing Office, 1979.

Public Knowledge

The public and high blood pressure: Six year followup survey of public knowledge and reported behavior (NIH Publication No. 81-2118). Washington, D.C.: U.S. Government Printing Office, 1981.

Physician Knowledge

Diagnosis and management of hypertension: A nationwide survey of physicians' knowledge, attitudes and reported behavior (USDHEW Publication No. [NIH] 79-1056). Washington, D.C.: U S. Government Printing Office, 1979.

General

Apostolides, A. Y., Oberman, A., Kraus, J. F., & Cutter, G. Impact of hypertension information on high blood pressure control between 1973 and 1978. *Hypertension,* 1980, *2,* 708–713.

Frommer, P. L., & Ward, G. W. Achievements and challenges in hypertension control. *Public Health Reports,* 1982, 97(2), inside cover.

Ward, G. W. Changing trends in hypertension control. *Public Health Reports,* 1978, *93*(1), 31–34.

Ward, G. W. The role of economic utilization and uncertainty. In P. D. Cooper, W. J. Kehoe, P. E. Murphy (Eds.), *Marketing and preventive health care: Interdisciplinary and interorganizational perspectives.* Chicago: American Marketing Association, 1978.

Ward, (W. Can preventive health care be marketed? Tailoring prevention to mass media. *American Pharmacy,* 1979, NS *19*(1), 11–13.

Ward, G. W., Morrison, W., & Schreiber, G. Pilot study of health professionals' awareness of the hypertension information in the mass media they use. *Public Health Reports,* 1982, 97(2), 113–115.

6

Social Marketing and Community Health Promotion

The Stanford Heart Disease Prevention Program

DOUGLAS S. SOLOMON

There is a long history of failure among social programs using mass media as their major sources of intervention. Health promotion programs, a subset of these social campaigns, have also failed to live up to their potential. In fact, a commonly held belief is that the mass media are impotent in changing health habits and promoting new health behaviors. Searching the literature on health promotion programs using mass media, one is at a loss to find more than a small handful of examples of campaigns that have even approximated their originally stated objectives. The *Stanford Heart Disease Prevention Program*'s (SHDPP) Three Community Study was initiated in 1972 to test, in realistic field settings, the potential for the use of community-based approaches in health promotion.

Novelli (1980) has summarized four basic problems in social campaigns. These include low visibility, low budgets, little research, and lack of continuity. Based on an understanding of these and other common problems in health promotion programs, the *Stanford Heart Disease Prevention Program* has utilized a vigorous social marketing perspective as one of its approaches in overcoming these major obstacles. This chapter will present an overview of the problem addressed by the SHDPP and

---

DOUGLAS S. SOLOMON • Formerly with the *Stanford Heart Disease Prevention Program,* Stanford University, Stanford, California; currently with Apple Computer, San Jose, California 95129. The studies reported on here were supported by NHLBI Grants #21906 (The Stanford Five City Multifactor Risk Reduction Study) and HL #14174 (The Stanford Specialized Center for Research in Arteriosclerosis).

describe the project from a social marketing perspective. Examples of particular applications of social marketing, including research techniques that have been used to design, implement, and monitor the progress of the education program, will be explored.

THE PROBLEM: HEART DISEASE

Cardiovascular disease is the greatest single killer of adults in the United States as well as in many other developed countries. The death rate due to heart disease has declined somewhat during the last decade in the United States and several other countries. However, heart disease is still responsible for the fact that the average U.S. male at age 40 has about the same life expectancy as the same-aged male at the turn of the century (U.S. Department of Health, Education, and Welfare, 1979).

There is much disagreement about the importance of various risk factors in heart disease. However, several studies have made it clear that smoking, high blood pressure, and high blood cholesterol are involved as risk factors (Truett, Cornfield, & Kannel, 1967; Intersociety Commission for Heart Disease Resources, Atherosclerosis Study Group, and Epidemiology Study Group, 1970). Other risk factors, including sedentary life-styles, overweight, stress, and dietary factors, are not at this point considered as important in terms of their evidence for contributing to heart disease, although they are still quite suspect. In an effort to understand the causes of heart disease, epidemiologists have observed that as life-style factors such as diet, stress, and physical activity vary among countries, so do cardiovascular disease rates. One example is an analysis comparing Japanese living in Japan to age-comparable Japanese Americans living in California (Robertson, Kelly, O'Neill, Wixom, Eisworth, & Haddon, 1974). Japanese in Japan have much lower death rates from heart disease than does the American sample, and Japanese who live in California have about the same rate of heart disease as other Americans. This indicates that as Japanese adopt various aspects of the American life-style, their disease rates tend to follow those of other Americans. It is therefore fairly widely accepted that although the exact contribution is not clear, many American life-style factors probably play an important role in cardiovascular disease rates. It has not been well demonstrated, however, that cardiovascular-disease-related morbidity or mortality can be reduced by changes in life-styles.

There are several current large-scale studies around the world designed to test the hypothesis that changing life-style factors can delay or prevent the onset of cardiovascular disease. One such study is being conducted by the SHDPP. Even with this background of the importance of heart disease prevention and some of the relevant factors related to heart disease, there are no well-developed techniques for changing risk factors. Even if current large-scale studies demonstrate that life-style factors are causally related to heart disease, there will still be no well-tested means to educate large numbers of individuals about the life-style changes needed to reduce risk in cost-effective ways. The SHDPP has been established to investigate the potential of large-scale prevention programs that can be implemented in a cost-effective manner. The approach chosen for testing in the SHDPP is a community-based approach.

There are many potential costs and benefits to using a community-based approach (Farquhar, 1978). One negative aspect of community-based approaches is a lesser degree of control over the content, frequency, and quality of health promotion messages than is possible in clinic-based or laboratory-based educational approaches. There are also some ethical problems inherent in educating entire communities without the consent of all of the individuals in them. However, it is the position of the SHDPP that these costs and others are far outweighed by the potential benefits. People live in communities. They interact with others. They are influenced by their friends, family, and peers. Therefore, the community setting offers many possible interactions due to interpersonal communication and influence patterns that are not generally available in a clinical setting. An additional benefit is that the mass media are available in community settings. Mass media have the ability to reach large numbers of people with high-frequency, high-quality messages at a low potential cost per unit of behavior change. Finally, it is certain that even if clinical approaches were perfected, there would be a huge lack of resources to provide these services to all individuals in the United States at risk of heart disease.

In summary, community-based approaches appear to have great potential for wide-scale, cost-effective prevention programs in heterogeneous free-living populations consisting of people who currently have heart disease, those who are at risk, and those who have not yet developed any relevant risk factors. The SHDPP was, therefore, established to test this kind of approach.

OVERVIEW OF THE *STANFORD HEART DISEASE PREVENTION PROGRAM*

On one hand, the SHDPP is a field experiment actually marketing heart disease prevention, and on the other hand, it is an experiment testing the efficacy of the process of changing risk factors on a wide variety of outcome measures. It may be useful to the reader to review briefly the objectives, design, and outcome of the SHDPP's two major community studies.

It should be said at the outset that the SHDPP is not a marketing project *per se.* Rather, it is an eclectic project drawing upon a large number of disciplines at many levels, including psychology, communication, community organization, and medicine as well as marketing. The SHDPP has been developed with an awareness of the best of what many disciplines, including marketing, have to offer. This chapter presents the program, however, within a marketing framework, in the hope that this mode of presentation will inform as well as stimulate the thinking of others working in similar areas of health promotion.

THE THREE COMMUNITY STUDY

The SHDPP began in 1970 with the formation of an interdisciplinary group of biomedical and behavioral science researchers determined to explore the potential of cardiovascular risk reduction through community education. This education would be administered primarily through the mass media in order to provide public health policymakers with information on the cost-effectiveness of community-wide public education.

In 1972, the Three Community Study began with funding from the National Heart, Lung, and Blood Institute of the National Institutes of Health. It was a quasi-experimental field study in three northern California towns. Two of the communities had extensive mass media campaigns over a 2-year period; in one of these the mass media were augmented with intensive face-to-face instruction of a small subset of individuals at high risk. The third community served as a control. This design was chosen in order to be able to contrast a lower cost mass media campaign using communication messages that focused on changing behavior patterns, compared to a much more expensive and labor-intensive mass media campaign supplemented with personal instruction. In this way, a potentially more cost-effective, generalizable approach could be compared to a more intensive and less generalizable model (Maccoby & Farquhar, 1975). People from each community were surveyed and examined for cardiovascular risk factors before the campaign began and at 1, 2, and 3 years afterward. Measurements were made of knowledge and behavior related to cardiovascular risk as well as physiological indicators of risk such as blood pressure, relative weight, and plasma cholesterol. In the community with both mass media and intensive instruction, the initial decrease in risk, as calculated by a multiple-logistic risk function (Truett *et al.*, 1967), was greater. By the second year, however, the mass-media-only community equaled it. Risk in the control community increased over the 2 years (Farquhar, Maccoby, Wood, Alexander, Breitrose, Brown, Haskell, McAlister, Meyer, Nash, & Stern, 1977; Maccoby, Farquhar, Wood, & Alexander, 1977). The results strongly suggested that mass media educational campaigns that are directed at entire communities can be effective in reducing the risk of heart attack and stroke. However, the results of the study pointed toward the importance of further research and development of methods to reduce smoking and increase physical activity using media alone.

From a marketing point of view, the Three Community Study was particularly important because, for virtually the first time, it had overcome many of the drawbacks and failures found in previous social campaigns (cf. Atkin, 1979; Novelli, 1980; Star & Hughes, 1950; Udry, 1974). In part, the original idea behind the

Three Community Study was sparked by a model developed by Cartwright (1949). Cartwright postulated that in order to modify behavior through mass media campaigns, three separate changes must be achieved: (1) changes in cognitive structures (i.e., what people know and understand), (2) changes in affective structures (i.e., what people want to do), and (3) changes in action structures (i.e., what people actually do and how this can be facilitated). In analyzing a campaign designed to encourage citizens to buy bonds during World War II, Cartwright found that traditional campaigns were usually successful in influencing information and attitudes (Steps 1 and 2 of his model) but were usually inadequate in promoting and guiding the specific actions advocated in the messages (Step 3). With Cartwright's model in mind, the SHDPP used mass media in a relatively novel way—using them to teach specific behavioral skills wherever possible. There is evidence that this approach worked. This perspective, adopted by the SHDPP, is very similar to a marketing orientation, particularly in terms of a concern for adequate mechanisms in communities (analogous to distribution channels) to ensure the availability and accessibility of change.

Maccoby and Alexander (1979) cited several other key features of the Three Community Study that were very similar to considerations found in typical marketing programs. These include (1) the establishment of specific objectives for each component of the campaign over time; (2) clearly defined audience segments; (3) the creation of clear, useful, and salient messages through formative research and pretesting; (4) utilization of creative media scheduling to reach the audience with adequate frequency; (5) stimulation of interpersonal communication to encourage a synergistic effect of multiple channels; (6) advocation of clear and well-paced behavioral changes in messages; (7) use of feedback to evaluate the campaign's progress over time; and (8) the use of a long-term campaign to avoid threshold effect considerations.

THE FIVE CITY PROJECT

The Three Community Study results prompted the design of a larger scale study that could implement recently developed and more effective behavior change strategies, focus more carefully on cost-effectiveness considerations, and include more extensive evaluation methods. This study, the Five City Project, began in the summer of 1978 (Maccoby & Solomon, 1981). Although it includes the successful elements of the previous study, it has been enlarged and improved. The new communities are much larger than the previous ones, the project will run from 5 to 8 years, community education efforts will be encouraged to continue indefinitely, and the sample of community participants is broadened to include all people from ages 12 to 74. The larger size of the communities and longer time span will enable the measurement of not only the risk of heart disease in individuals, but they will make it possible to detect differences in cardiovascular morbidity and mortality rates in the communities. Finally, the most important aspect of the current project is its emphasis on generalizability and cost-effectiveness. A major goal is to develop a model program that can be adopted by other communities. Because of this concern for generalizability, Stanford's direct involvement in the community education program has been limited to encourage the widest possible participation of local groups, a potentially cost-effective and generalizable approach.

In summary, from a social marketing point of view, some unique elements of the SHDPP Five City Project stand out. It is highly research oriented, and at the same time it is action oriented. Formative research is a formal component of the project process. It is used for decision making and management purposes as well as for monitoring the progress and pitfalls of the campaign. Secondly, it is highly cost conscious and concerned with generalizability.

The midrange goals of the SHDPP Five City Project after 2 years of educational activity include significant reductions in cardiovascular risk that should, after 8 years, lead to significant reductions in morbidity and mortality. For the education communities as a whole, the goal is a net reduction (in comparison to the control communities) in tobacco use, body weight, blood pressure, and cholesterol that will lead to a reduction in overall risk of cardiovascular disease in the area of 20%.

MARKET ANALYSES

In order to analyze the market for risk reduction in the target communities, one of the initial steps in the Five City Project was an ambitious baseline survey. Other methods have also been utilized for the market analysis, including unobtrusive measures, secondary data analyses, and much market research that we call *formative research*. These methods, particularly formative research, will be described in a subsequent section of this chapter. As the name suggests, the Five City Project is being conducted in five California communities, each of moderate size, that vary in population from 44,000 to 130,000. Four of the communities have survey centers established for baseline and subsequent surveys. All five communities are monitored for morbidity and mortality using an innovative surveillance system. Two of the five communities are receiving the education program, whereas the others are comparison communities. The permanent survey center established in each of the four communities is staffed by a nurse supervisor, an interviewer/abstractor, a laboratory technician, and a medical office assistant. Using letters as well as interpersonal communication approaches, the staff members invited a random sample of households to visit the survey center for a comprehensive evaluation prior to the start of education. In the first year of the survey, roughly 600 people in each of the four communities visited the survey centers. This comprised the first independent sample. After about 1 year, these same individuals were invited to return to the survey centers for a follow-up evaluation. They will be evaluated every other year for 6 years and constitute a cohort sample. This cohort sample has been established in order to study the process of change in risk and behavior in individuals. This procedure should provide valuable knowledge on individual change processes that can be only studied using a cohort sample. In order to avoid the bias inherent in cohort samples, independent samples are also used to study cross-sections of the community over time. These independent samples are being selected from the communities and interviewed every other year during the course of the project. Only the baseline survey will be discussed here, because it was used for planning purposes as well as for summative evaluation.

The baseline survey consisted of four main components: the core questionnaire, the formative questionnaire, physiological measures, and biochemical tests. This survey required about 2 hr of participant time. The goal of the core questionnaire was to provide a baseline for use in planning as well as in subsequent measures of change processes related to cardiovascular risk, knowledge, attitudes, and behavior. It consisted of 10 sections: demographic measures; attitude and opinion measures; health knowledge assessment related to heart disease, stroke, and various preventive measures; stress behavior; diet/nutrition and weight behavior; smoking behavior; physical activity behavior; communication media use and interpersonal communication patterns; community organization memberships and involvement and an interpersonal communication network analysis; and medical history including medication use. Finally, a random 40% of the participants was administered a 24-hr dietary recall measure in order to gather data on their food consumption. The other 60% was administered a series of formative evaluation questionnaires. The physiological measures included resting heart rate, blood pressure, height and weight, and a low-level fitness test using a calibrated stationary bicycle. Biochemical tests included urinary sodium, potassium, and creatinine; blood lipids; carbon monoxide concentration in expired air; and serum thiocyanate (an unobtrusive measure of smoking).

This survey, which was obviously quite extensive, provided no major surprises in terms of the overall planning process. The results of the survey, as was expected from our analysis of national data, found that there was considerable risk in the study communities as there is in most American communities. This was known before the study was planned in order to justify the funding of such a comprehensive field experiment. However, at another level, the formative uses of the data for planning purposes and the formative questionnaires themselves provided much useful, interesting, and unexpected results as input to the planning process.

DEVELOPING THE PROGRAM

A heart disease prevention program consists of a number of somewhat independent but interacting programs on risk factors such as smoking, weight loss, nutrition, high blood pressure, and stress. Each of these risk factors may be present in various types of individuals at various points in their lives. Some people are aware and concerned about their risk, whereas others are not. Therefore, the conduct of such a broad campaign requires careful focusing of efforts and planning. The initial approach used in planning the SHDPP Five City Project was to create overall objectives and a rationale for achieving these objectives. Based on the behavioral objectives for each of the risk factors, which were set in order to accomplish statistically significant as well as meaningful outcomes, we formed expert groups. These expert groups, centered around each of the risk factor areas, were given the task of creating a planning guide that would specify, based on the current state of the art, specific target audiences for each of these risk factor behavior change goals and how best to accomplish these goals. Sometimes, prefield investigations were necessary in particular areas that had very little existing research in order to test various approaches to change. For example, the SHDPP conducted a prefield study on approaches to smoking prevention programs among teenagers. Concurrent with the planning, meetings were conducted with community leaders to engage their participation in the program and to begin to develop contacts in each of the communities among local groups, health professionals, individuals, and the mass media.

Based on all these analyses and planning activities, we developed a series of "waves" that would focus the activities of the education program on particular risk factor areas at certain points in time. The first wave was on general risk reduction and included the production and airing of a 1-hr TV special, "The Heart Health Test." This program was designed to provide information to individuals about risk factors, stimulate their interests in reducing risk, teach relevant skills, and provide some awareness of the existence of the SHDPP within the communities. Formative research was used to design the TV presentation as well as to evaluate its impact.

Subsequent waves of the campaign focused on areas such as smoking cessation and nutrition. Each wave was planned by first considering the ultimate objectives at the end of the 5-year education program, then by working backward and determining how much change must occur each year in the risk factors to meet these goals. Based on research identifying who is at risk for each factor (e.g., which market segment), various programs and activities were planned that were based on what would appeal to the individuals at risk and what would have a high probability of achieving successful risk reduction. This goal-oriented planning process started with ultimate objectives and worked back to interim objectives and alternative approaches to reaching particular audience segments. This is a difficult process because data are not always available on the efficacy of various approaches or on particular needs or desires of certain target groups. Decisions were made in a pragmatic fashion considering the potential payoff of each approach based on whatever data were available regarding the efficacy of each approach. At the same time, it was necessary to consider the need to create lasting relationships between the project and the ultimate consumers as well as intermediaries such as community groups, health professionals, and the mass media. Often, data are simply not available on the efficacy of a given approach, and decisions must be made based on face validity, prefield experiments, and intuition. In every case, these programs are intensely evaluated in order to provide subsequent information on their effectiveness for future use.

To provide a slightly more structured approach to the development and implementation of the education program, it may be useful to present it from the point of view of the four *p*'s of marketing—product, price, place, and promotion. After these are described, additional information will be presented on actual projects that have required marketing decision making and implementation using marketing approaches. Particular emphasis will be placed on formative research and analysis as used within the Five City Project.

One overall planning framework has been very useful in the design of the Five City Project products and promotional strategies. This framework is called the hierarchy of effects framework (HEF) and has been described elsewhere in various forms by McGuire (1969), Rogers and Shoemaker (1971), and several other authors. An example of this framework related to heart disease is illustrated in Figure 1. This hierarchy of effects example assumes that individuals proceed through various steps during the process of change. They do not necessarily experience all of them or in the same order but, in general, these steps include awareness, knowledge, motivation, skills learning, action/behavior, and maintenance of behavior change. Even though each of these steps may not be relevant for a given behavioral domain, they provide a useful framework for examining the potential needs for changing behavior in each area. Figure 1 shows which steps in each of the risk factors described are generally lacking in the Five City Project audience. For example, formative research in the area of smoking cessation shows that there is much awareness, some knowledge, and strong motivation (because many people have tried to quit smoking many times but failed). Yet, there is a lack of skills related to being able to successfully quit smoking and a lack of strategies for maintaining that kind of behavior. One can see in the

		RISK FACTORS			
		SMOKING	EXERCISE	STRESS	NUTRITION
STAGES IN A BEHAVIOR CHANGE PROCESS	AWARENESS	+	+	+	+
	KNOWLEDGE	+	—	—	—
	MOTIVATION	+	+	+	—
	SKILLS LEARNING	—	—	—	—
	MAINTENANCE AND SELF MANAGEMENT	—	—	—	—

Figure 1. Hierarchy of effects framework in heart disease prevention.

other risk factors the behavioral areas that are present or lacking. By examining each risk factor for each audience segment using this type of hierarchy, the SHDPP is able to plan its products and promotional strategies. In this way, it is possible to deal educationally with levels of the hierarchy that are lacking rather than areas that may be already present or irrelevant to achieving behavior change. For example, smoking prevention and cessation programs for many years focused only at the knowledge and awareness levels, informing the audience of the health hazards of smoking and smoking's connections with heart disease and cancer. However, based on our analysis, this kind of approach should not be the major one at this time. Therefore, we choose to focus on other areas that have a greater probability of completing a hierarchy of effects and leading to behavior change. With this hierarchy of effects framework in mind, we proceed now to describe the four *p*'s of marketing as they relate to the SHDPP.

The Product

The word *product* is used here to refer to both products (such as a heart-healthy cookbook) as well as services (such as a smoking cessation class). A product (or service) is defined as the focus of the transaction that takes place in marketing between the marketer and the target audience. The core generic product of the SHDPP is improved information, motivation, and skills training on how to quit smoking, how and why to lose weight, how to reduce stress, how to increase physical activity, and how to prepare healthier meals. The SHDPP has a highly complex and large product line. Various products are oriented toward different target audiences. For example, information for youth is very different than that for adults. Special informational materials and other products are prepared for health professionals that will not be available to the other segments. Different kinds of information products are created in Spanish rather than in English, reflecting the particular culture and needs of each group.

Although our core product is information, it comes in many different forms. Some information is transmitted over the electronic media and is therefore intangible; other information exists in tangible form such as books, booklets, and video and audiotape cassettes. These products must all be carefully conceptualized, designed, and marketed. Another key product class in the SHDPP is the programs that are presented through the auspices of existing community organizations such as stop-smoking programs, nutrition and weight loss programs, and exercise programs.

The formative research and planning process contributes to the careful conceptualization and design of these products. Some examples of how formative research has contributed to the product design process include the design of the "Healthy Living" series of viodetapes and the *Heart Health Tip Sheets*. The tip sheets are a series of 12 printed 8½ in. × 11 in. sheets of paper that provide information to people in small, digestible bits. The idea for the tip sheets grew out of a formative research study on print materials. In this study, a hypothesis about refrigerators' being a major information center in the home was tested. It was found that the majority of refrigerators have information on them, including much information about health and nutrition. Furthermore, it was found that magnets, particularly those in the shape of butterflies, hold up most of this material. Therefore, this research confirmed the initial creative idea of the SHDPP print media director, and the tip sheet project was born. The tip sheets were direct mailed, one every 2 weeks, with a heart-shaped magnet displaying the SHDPP logo to hold them on the refrigerator door. They were very well accepted, and follow-up studies have shown that they were utilized by recipients far more than the majority of health information materials.

The "Healthy Living" series has grown out of a need expressed by the SHDPP communities for information on risk factor reduction that is neatly packaged and can be used over and over again in group settings. Rather than necessitating a highly trained discussion leader, it was decided that the bulk of the information could be packaged into short, 15–20 min videotapes. A pilot test of the series is being formatively evaluated in order to provide information for future versions of it. Other products of the SHDPP that have grown out of formative evaluation and other kinds of feedback include a weight-loss correspondence course and a do-it-yourself quit-smoking kit.

Throughout all of these discussions about the SHDPP's product line, the common theme is a concern for products oriented not only toward the key target groups but also to secondary groups such as health professionals, community organizations, and individuals. These products have grown out of formative research and intensive interactions with the communities. An example of current formative research is a study of physicians that is being done in order to assess their health-education-oriented attitudes, practices, and perceptions of needs for patient education materials.

The Place

As with the products, the distribution channels used are highly diversified, depending on the specific product to be distributed and the target audience. In general, the distribution channels include (1) the mass media (including radio, television, newspapers, booklets, and posters), (2) health professionals (including continuing education programs for health professionals at all levels and distribution of health information through health professional's work places), (3) community organizations (such as heart and lung associations, health departments, fraternal and youth organizations), and (4) commercial channels (such as bookstores, drugstores, and grocery stores).

In terms of the mass media, most of the distribution has been conducted as a public service of the mass media themselves. This is probably one of the few generalizable models of health promotion because purchasing media time and space is extremely expensive. All of our radio and television programs have been broadcast during public service time. Although it is often a problem to obtain sufficient public service time, particularly time other than in the early morning hours, our project has been highly successful in achieving prime time distribution of messages through the development of special relationships with the mass media outlets. These special relationships have grown out of the mass media gatekeepers' understanding of the importance of our program and of their having a cooperative relationship with us that we have developed over time. They are considered full partners in the educational process and are therefore quite happy to present jointly designed educational materials that are well developed and tested for their particular audiences.

Health professionals, ranging from physical activity teachers and physical therapists to nurses and doctors, are distributors in several ways. One major way is by informing them about our health promotion messages so that they can pass these on to their patients and clients. Health professionals are also quite interested in distributing SHDPP's printed and other materials. In fact, we are in the process of designing materials specifically for distribution by health professionals. In the past year we have pilot tested a physician pad that can be used to record each patient's blood pressure and given to the patient to facilitate the education of what blood pressure is and what patients can do about it. This is currently being evaluated using a mail and telephone survey in order to determine its effectiveness and its implications for future use.

Community organizations have been widely involved in the distribution process. For example, we have worked intensively with the county health department to provide classes on smoking cessation. The *Weight Loss by Mail* program is being distributed through a local community college. A large local employer is distributing educational messages through its newsletter to Spanish-speaking employees.

Commercial channels are a promising source of distribution, however, they have not been heavily utilized up to this point. One way they have been utilized is through the sale of some of our booklets, which are being distributed by a commercial book and magazine dealer in the communities. Several drugstores are also distributing printed materials as their form of cooperation with the program. Some commercial organizations have chosen to sponsor television programs, assisting us in this manner to distribute health messages to individuals.

Our concern with distribution is to provide the audience with multiple opportunities, places, and forms for achieving self-directed behavior change. They can choose to make changes on their own or in some organized program. This can be done with or without our printed and audiovisual materials. The key is to offer a choice of multiple channels with the assumption that different people are likely to desire and to select different alternatives and that the availability of one alternative augments that of another. This diversity of channels is one important component contributing to what is planned to be a synergistic campaign effect.

Much formative research is devoted to determining the best distribution channels for given messages on various risk factors. For example, in our analysis of the potential for smoking cessation programs, we analyzed memberships in community organizations within the group of smokers and found that organizations such as veterans and fraternal organizations had a very high proportion of smokers. In the youth area, we analyzed which grades smokers were enrolled in and in which grades students begin experimenting with smoking to determine some intervention points in the school system. This understanding of where the audience is in terms of physical location, group membership, and mass media use is very important in designing an optimal distribution strategy.

The Price

The price of participation in risk reduction activities includes time, social support, psychological, and monetary costs. Because of this complexity and the high degree of integration of costs with the design of the product itself, it is difficult to discuss the price factor separately. However, through our formative research program, we are investigating many of these cost factors. For example, our survey of risk-related attitudes includes a fairly comprehensive section that deals with the psychological costs (and benefits) of changing one's health behavior. We also are studying in detail the costs, in terms of social support, of entering into some kind of organized program or even of changing health behavior on an individual basis. For example, we find that smokers who live with other smokers may require different programs than those who live in nonsmoking households. Additionally, we are carefully studying psychological and monetary cost factors related to joining various kinds of self-change programs. This includes studying the specific places where people would like to attend programs (i.e., the YMCA as compared to the community college), the sources of the program (i.e., conducted by an expert leader or by a lay person), the kinds of people involved, and the sizes of the groups. These data can be used to develop a plan for an optimal stop-smoking or weight loss program for various segments of the audience.

For example, we found that two-thirds of all smokers in our survey preferred to quit smoking on their own and not in a group setting, and 21% were interested in using self-help materials. These results suggest different audience segments based on the varying psychological and other costs associated with each cessation method. Research is also being conducted on the optimal price to charge for classes based on what people can afford to pay, so as not to exclude them because of their income, as well as a recognition that price sometimes carries with it a meaning of quality. In our sample, 56% of the smokers would be willing to pay $100 or less for a class, 21% would pay from $100 to $300, and 23% would pay more than $300 if they thought the class would enable them to quit smoking. Similar analyses of cost factors have also been conducted in the exercise area. As was mentioned in the section on distribution, our policy is to offer choices of various products. This implies a product line with variously priced products. Someone who wants to learn to quit smoking can join a smoking cessation class at relatively high time costs (even though no money is charged). Others may prefer to use a copy of our do-it-yourself quit-smoking tip sheet kit, and still others may prefer to watch our TV series on the local news show at very low psychological, monetary, time, and social costs.

The Promotion

Promotion within the context of a social-marketing-oriented program is somewhat different than promotion within a commercial program. In commercial programs, promotion usually includes advertising, sales promotion, and public relations related to the tangible products sold by a particular commercial concern. In a project such as the SHDPP in which many products are intangible and consist mainly of information, promotion plays a slightly different role. We use advertisements, for example, not to promote anything else but to provide information. These have already been described under the product section because we consider them to be products of our program. Nevertheless, both mass media products as well as community events benefit from promotion. For mass media products we utilize multiple channels to accomplish this goal.

An example of our approach to promotion is the "Heart Health Test," a 1-hr TV special produced by the SHDPP, which was aired in prime time to provide information and some skills training on heart disease risk reduction. After the first broadcast, we conducted a follow-up telephone survey that asked questions related to how people had heard about the program. We used this information to design the promotion for the second airing of this program a year later. We then conducted a field experiment to test the relative effectiveness of several alternative promotion approaches. The major approach tested was the use of direct mail flyers in order to encourage people to watch the show. A random sample of the community was chosen and half were sent a flyer describing the program and providing them with a score card for the test itself. Subsequent to showing the TV special, a follow-up telephone survey was conducted to determine the effectiveness of this direct mail promotion. It was found that 22% watched the program who had not received the direct mail promotion and that 31% watched the program who had received the direct mail. This showed that direct mail significantly increased ($p \leq .05$) the audience of the television show. Other approaches used to promote the show included encouraging schoolchildren to watch the show by distributing letters to their teachers and asking the children to encourage their parents to watch the show. This was evaluated through a survey of teachers. A final method of promotion that was tested included asking community groups to encourage their members to watch.

Another common method we use to promote products is through the newspaper. For example, after a recently published exercise booklet was promoted in our weekly newspaper doctors' column, we immediately received several hundred telephone requests for copies. Promotion of media programs and products is a very difficult and time-consuming task. Therefore, as can be seen in the previous examples, the SHDPP is attempting to evaluate various approaches to promotion in order to determine the most cost-effective and reliable methods.

Similarly, community events such as fun runs, smoking classes, weight loss programs, and lectures are promoted, using a combination of media and interpersonal communication. These are being constantly evaluated in order to provide implications for future promotions. One method we have established for evaluating promotion is to use a standardized form that we ask participants in group events to fill out. This form asks them to report how they heard about the program, whether through interpersonal or mass media sources or both. In this way, we will be able to determine the channels that have most effectively contributed to awareness and participation in community events. Other methods used to evaluate community event promotions include such things as telephone surveys and the major summative surveys that continuously monitor how people heard about and what motivated them to attend community events.

FORMATIVE RESEARCH'S ROLE IN THE SHDPP

Social marketing practice, to a large degree, is based on formative research. *Formative research* is defined as any research designed to provide guidance for educational planners in facilitating the development of appropriate, attractive, and effective educational and community programs. The SHDPP's integrated formative research component has five basic purposes.

1. The collection of baseline data for developing audience profiles and for defining specific subaudiences called market segments. This research attempts to answer questions related to what people are like in terms of their needs, their desires, their priorities, and their past experiences related to risk reduction.
2. Collection of information for specific program planning (e.g., Which of the following five smoking cessation programs would you most like to participate in? What are the attributes of attractive physical activity programs for various audience segments?).
3. Collection of information for specific media programs (the design of attrac-

tive, interesting, and useful booklets, TV spots, posters, etc.). This research attempts to package media products so that they provide the intended information and encourage the intended behavior changes in ways that attract people's attention and active participation.

4. Process analysis of media events. Process analysis is research designed to determine whether or not educational programs are meeting interim, short-range goals. If they do not meet interim goals, it is very unlikely they will meet their ultimate goals. Therefore, process research studies provide interim goal attainment measures necessary to diagnose possible successes or failures in media events. An example of this is a study to determine how many people recall receiving a booklet sent to them in the mail, how many remember the title, say they read it and learned anything from it. If these interim goals are not achieved, it is unlikely that this booklet will lead to risk factor reduction.
5. Process analysis of educational programs. This is the analog of process analysis for media events and includes such things as: Have you heard about our exercise groups? Have you participated in smoking groups? What do you think of your experience in our weight loss program?

The sources of information for formative research include both the baseline surveys and subsequent follow-up surveys (which are intended mainly as summative research) and special formative questionnaires administered at baseline and subsequent surveys. Many special studies are done periodically to gather specific information using techniques such as telephone interviews, personal interviews, and shopping center intercept surveys.

The formative questionnaires used in the surveys were designed to progress in a series of waves over time. This was done for several reasons. One reason was that formative data do not need to be as precise in terms of statistical confidence as summative data because the goal of formative research is usually to know the range of opinions on an issue rather than having accurate estimates of proportions responding in one way or another. Second, there were many more formative questions at baseline that needed asking than could be asked of any given participant at any time. Therefore, four waves of formative questionnaires were designed and implemented on various random subsamples of the baseline population before the beginning of the SHDPP education program in April 1980. These waves included the following:

1. *General health perceptions and motivations.* This is a questionnaire designed to provide information on people's own health priorities and desires for personal change, their motivations for changing, and some ideas about potential blockages to change.
2. *Nutrition and weight loss material design and marketing.* This questionnaire provided information on behavior related to eating, such as food shopping behavior, food preparation behavior, decision making about foods within

households, information on past experiences with various kinds of weight loss programs, and information related to print materials, including data on where people buy print materials on health, the kinds of materials they own, and implications for the design of a most desirable cookbook.

3. *Print preferences and strategy testing*. This questionnaire provided guidance for the development of a booklet that was published during the Five City Project. It also tested hypotheses on various information delivery systems that led, as has been previously described, to the design and implementation of refrigerator tip sheets.
4. *Physical activity, stress, and weight loss program design*. This questionnaire gathered information related to designing programs such as the most desired kinds of physical activities, places, and times desired for physical activity programs and also dealt with the semantics of heart disease in an attempt to learn the meanings people attach to words that can be used to describe various elements of heart disease prevention. For example, it is important to avoid using words that are negatively loaded, and it is important to use words that people understand and are comfortable with.

This formative data bank is providing valuable information at many different levels for the planning of the SHDPP educational program. These levels include simply knowing the words people use to describe various risk factors; content analysis of questions people have about various risk factors that we can use to infer the ways that they categorize this information; and specific questions, comments, attitudes, and ideas people have about optimal risk reduction programs. Subsequent to these four waves of formative data collection, which continue to provide useful information, we have conducted many content analysis studies and other kinds of message and product design studies to help in the educational design and implemen-

Table 1. Examples of SHDPP Formative Research

- Risk factor analyses of baseline summative data on nutrition, weight, exercise, and smoking
- Analysis of questions people have about nutrition, exercise, and weight control
- Semantic differential tests of words associated with physical activity
- Pretest of the questions to be used in the "Heart Health Test" TV show
- Follow-up ratings survey on viewers of the "Heart Health Test"
- Pretest of the do-it-yourself smoking tip sheet quit kit
- SHDPP logo recognition (and meaning attributed to it) survey
- Test of three heart magnets to choose the optimal one for gaining name recognition
- Pretest of eight TV spots on smoking cessation
- Pretest of four TV spots on nutrition
- Evaluations of all major classes, including smoking cessation and "Healthy Living" classes
- Survey of physicians receiving the MD blood pressure information pads
- Survey of physicians on needs for patient education materials
- Field study on the promotional methods used for the "Heart Health Test"

tation. The formative research methods used are almost identical to those used in summative research and include surveys, individual interviews, focus group discussions, field experiments, as well as unobtrusive measures. We have also done much analysis of the baseline summative data for formative purposes, such as analyses of smoker's knowledge, attitudes, and behaviors, and knowledge, attitudes, and behaviors related to weight loss, nutrition, exercise, and blood pressure. Some examples of formative research projects that have been conducted are shown in Table 1.

RESULTS AND IMPLICATIONS

Results

Although the first follow-up study of the original survey cohort has recently been completed, the results are not yet available for publication. Therefore, it is impossible to assess at this point the impact of the Five City Project on risk-related knowledge, attitudes, and behavior. However, because of the formative process analysis that has been conducted, it is possible to make guesses about the probable impact. We have seen that most of the educational materials have been well accepted and utilized by the community. The mass media programs have received ratings comparable to other prime time radio and television programming. We have received many requests for printed materials based on media promotions and have seen much community awareness and requests from the community for the development of further programming. Therefore, we are optimistic that the process is achieving interim goals and will continue to be successful and ultimately lead to the desired mortality and morbidity changes.

There are basically three factors in planning social campaigns such as the SHDPP that probably account for the success or failure of these programs. They have been described elsewhere in detail (Maccoby & Solomon, 1981) and include four key areas: problem analysis and strategy design, media selection, message and community program design, and evaluation research. Social marketing philosophy, strategies, and techniques play a large role in optimizing each of these areas of social campaign design. Formative research, in particular, is critical to each of these areas. *Problem analysis and strategy design* is a process of refining the overall goals of an education program based on much analysis and some minimal formative research. The goal of problem analysis is to create objectives that are specific, measurable, and achievable. These objectives usually define goals in terms of specific outcomes, such as knowledge change, attitude change, behavioral intention change, and various target behavior changes. Formative research and other kinds of market research techniques are useful in the problem, definition, and analysis processes.

Media selection is a process of defining which media, including mass and interpersonal communication media, are best matched with the particular goals of each component of the campaign. Market research techniques are very useful in choosing media and group settings that are attractive to people and that will encourage much needed participation.

Message and program design is the process of setting specific subobjectives for each message or program and generating alternative approaches, pretesting them, and revising them before implementation so that they can meet their original objectives. Although community program design is relatively lacking in theory and past research, message design is based on a great treasurehouse of research into key variables such as sources, channels, and receivers (cf. McGuire, 1981; Schramm; 1972; Zimbardo, Ebbesen, & Maslach, 1977).

Finally, *evaluation research* is the key area often neglected in campaigns. Campaigns at times simply ignore evaluation or ask questions related only to whether or not the campaign succeeded or failed. Ignoring the process analysis of a campaign usually provides no information to subsequent planners on the reasons for success or failure of a past effort. Therefore, formative research using marketing techniques such as those used in the Five City Project can provide this needed process analysis that can change the direction of a project while being implemented. It can also provide meaningful information for subsequent planners in similar content areas. It is important for health promotion project planners to consider these four key concerns of health promotion in order to maximize their potential impact and to understand the process of change associated with their programs.

Another part of this planning process that is a critical aspect of social marketing is the importance of having realistic criteria for success in health promotion programs. Social marketing suggests that expectations for success should be similar to those evidenced in commercial marketing programs. These expectations are typically quite minimal and may seem too small for those engaged in social pursuits. However, these expectations are generally based on data related to the potential audience, the audience's potential willingness to change, and the potential effects of given interventions. The kind of thinking that looks into these factors in the prediction of success is a very important addition to the planning evident in most health promotion and other social programs. In reviewing virtually all past health campaigns, Atkin (1979) made a point of stressing that expectation of success should not be exaggerated and should be based on data, including formative research.

Implications

In looking toward the future of health promotion programs, it is clear that social marketing is going to play a much greater role. Fox and Kotler (1980, p. 32) have documented the growth of social marketing in its first 10 years. They firmly believe that "social marketing specialists, combining business marketing skills with additional training in the social sciences, will be working on a wider range of social causes with increasing sophistication."

There are five key areas of social marketing influence that may play this critical role in the future of health promotion programs. The first is encouraging explicit definitions of goals and objectives. Health promotion programs, if they are to be successful, must move away from broad definitions to very specific, operational definitions that can be evaluated. Second, social marketing experts will encourage health promotion programs to know audience characteristics, needs, attitudes, and desires, and to use these as "guiding lights" for developing and implementing programs. This will avoid the previous mentality, called by marketing experts a *sales mentality,* in which those designing programs think they know best what people should be told and how they should be told it. In particular, where there is competition in health programs with commercial concerns, this knowledge of audience characteristics and desires will be critical in achieving success. Third, there will be an increasing use of audience segmentation strategies, such as those evidenced in the SHDPP, in health promotion programs. Health programs will move away from the previous emphasis on being all things to all people and increasingly turn toward specific subaudiences and each group's specific need. This will increase their probability for success. Fourth, health promotion programs will depend more and more on formative research for planning and program monitoring processes. In this way, they will be able to avoid a sales mentality and achieve their audience segmentation based on research. Finally, like marketing programs, health promotion programs will be concerned with the use of local resources and cost-effectiveness expertise so that programs will be effective as well as manageable in terms of their overall costs to individuals and to society. The use of existing commercial resources and community resources that have long been ignored by social programs may become an important characteristic in the future.

SUMMARY

Heart disease is a major public health problem in the United States as well as in many other countries. Currently, however, there are no well-tested techniques for changing individuals' risk factor status on a large-scale basis. The *Stanford Heart Disease Prevention Program*'s Five City Project is designed to test the hypothesis that reducing life-style factors can delay or prevent cardiovascular disease. Its community-based approach may well be one of the only cost-effective and generalizable models for ameliorating a wide range of public health problems. The SHDPP utilizes a variety of theoretical frameworks and, in particular, a social marketing framework for planning and implementation processes. Marketing-oriented research serves as a major force in the planning process and has set the course for many of the SHDPP's community and mass media programs.

The core product of the SHDPP is information in a wide variety of forms. Information packages are developed based on a clear understanding of the needs, past experiences, knowledge levels, attitudes, and behavioral skills of a wide variety of audience segments. The major distribution channels of the program include health professionals, mass media, community groups, and commercial channels. A particular emphasis is placed on the cost of changing health habits from an individual and community psychological as well as monetary point of view. The promotional strategies of the SHDPP are widely varied and include the use of mass media as well as community resources. Formative research, which is analogous to marketing research, serves as a key role in optimizing the four *p*'s of marketing within the context of the SHDPP.

In summary, from a social marketing point of view, the SHDPP utilizes several key elements that are unique to many health programs. These include a reliance on formative research, extensive use of audience segmentation, development of multiple products that are targeted to each primary and secondary audience, a concern for the price of engaging in risk reduction behaviors from an individual point of view, and a distribution system that utilizes existing channels for cost-effectiveness and external generalizability.

Although there is obviously no guarantee that this approach will be successful in meeting its objectives, it nevertheless uses the best planning frameworks available and will provide a significant test of a model that can ultimately, if successful, be realistically applied to the improvement of health conditions in entire communities in the United States and throughout the world. Future improvements of many health conditions may rely on this type of community-based, low-cost approach.

REFERENCES

Atkin, C. K. Research evidence on mass mediated health communication campaigns. *Communication yearbook 3*. New Brunswick, N.J.: Transaction Books, 1979.

Cartwright, D. Some principles of mass persuasion: Selected findings of research on the sale of U.S. war bonds. In W. Schramm & D. Roberts (Eds.), *The process and effects of mass communication* (2nd ed.). Champaign: University of Illinois Press, 1949.

Farquhar, J. W., Maccoby, N., Alexander, J., Breitrose, H., Brown, B., Haskell, W., McAlister, A., Meyer, A., Nash, J., & Stern, M. Community education for cardiovascular health. *The Lancet*, 1977, *1*, 1192–1195.

Farquhar, J. W. The community-based models of life-style intervention trials. *American Journal of Epidemiology*, 1978, *108*, 103–111.

Fox, K., & Kotler, P. The marketing of social causes: The first 10 years. *Journal of Marketing*, 1980, *44*, 24–33.

Intersociety Commission for Heart Disease Resources, Atherosclerosis Study Group, and Epidemiology Study Group. Primary prevention of the atherosclerotic disease. *Circulation*, 1970, *42*, 42–45.

Maccoby, N., & Alexander, J. Use of media in life-style programs. In P. Davidson (Ed.), *Behavior medicine: Changing health life styles*. Calgary, Alberta, Canada: Banff International Conferences on Behavior Modification, 1979.

Maccoby, N., & Farquhar, J. Communication for health: Unselling heart disease. *Journal of Communication,* 1975, *25,* 114–126.

Maccoby, N., & Solomon, D. Heart disease prevention: Community studies. In R. Rice & W. Paisley (Eds.), *Public communication campaigns.* Beverly Hills, Cal.: Sage Publications, 1981.

Maccoby, N., Farquhar, J., Wood, P., & Alexander, J. Reducing the risk of cardiovascular disease: Effect of a community-based campaign on knowledge and behavior. *Journal of Community Health,* 1977, *3,* 100–114.

McGuire, W. J. The nature of attitudes and attitude change. In G. Lindzey & E. Aronson (Eds.), *The handbook of social psychology.* Menlo Park, Cal.: Addison-Wesley, 1969.

McGuire, W. J. Theoretical foundation of campaigns. In R. Rice & W. Paisley (Eds.), *Public communication campaigns.* Beverly Hills, Cal.: Sage Publications, 1981.

Novelli, W. Confessions of a social marketer. In K. Fox & P. Kotler (Chairs), *Social marketing in action.* Symposium presented at the meetings of the American Marketing Association, Chicago, August 1980.

Robertson, L. S., Kelley, A. B., O'Neill, B., Wixom, C. W., Eisworth, R. S., & Haddon, W. Epidemiology of coronary heart disease and stroke in Japanese men living in Japan, Hawaii, and California. *American Journal of Public Health,* 1974, *64,* 1071–1080.

Rogers, E., with Shoemaker, F. *Communication of innovations: A cross-cultural approach.* New York: Free Press, 1971.

Schramm, W. What the research says. In Wilbur Schramm (Ed.), *Quality in instructional television.* Honolulu: The University Press of Hawaii, 1972.

Star, S., & Hughes, H. A report on an educational campaign: The Cincinnati plan for the United Nations. *American Journal of Sociology,* 1950, *55,* 389–400.

Truett, J., Cornfield, J., & Kannel, W. A multivariate analysis of the risk of coronary heart disease in Framingham. *Journal of Clinical Disorders,* 1967, *20,* 511–524.

U.S. Department of Health, Education, and Welfare. *Healthy people: Surgeon general's report on health promotion and disease prevention.* Washington, D.C.: Government Printing Office, 1979.

Udry, J. R. *The mass media and family planning.* New York: Ballinger, 1974.

Zimbardo, P., Ebbesen, E., & Maslach, C. *Influencing attitudes and changing behavior.* Menlo Park, Cal.: Addison-Wesley, 1977.

7

Marketing Health to Employees

The Johnson & Johnson Live for Life™ *Program*

CURTIS S. WILBUR and DAVID GARNER

THE PROBLEM

A growing consensus within the biomedical, academic, and government communities developed in the late 1970s that individual life-styles were a prominent factor in the major causes of premature death and disability. Smoking, poor diet, lack of regular exercise, and poor stress management were linked to cardiovascular disease and cancer, the cause of 75% of all deaths within the United States. Moreover, preliminary results from such programs as the Stanford Three Community Study and the North Karelia Project suggested that the life-styles of large numbers of people could be altered through community-wide interventions. Clearly, the opportunity existed to prevent or reduce the premature occurrence of life-style disease.

At the same time, financial pressure was building to act on skyrocketing illness-care costs (broadly defined as costs incurred due to hospitalization, medical, dental, short- and long-term disability, sick days, workman's compensation, and life insurance). Like many major business corporations, Johnson & Johnson is self-insured for employee and dependent illness-care costs. By the mid 1970s, these costs were no longer an insignificant part of a comprehensive employee benefits package. The accelerating illness-care costs seen nationally ($229 billion in 1980 and estimated to be $450 billion by 1985) were also keenly felt at Johnson & Johnson. Since 1977, Johnson & Johnson illness-care costs have increased at an annual rate of 19%.

CURTIS S. WILBUR and DAVID GARNER • *Live for Life* Program, Johnson & Johnson, New Brunswick, New Jersey 08903.

In 1980, illness costs alone represented 2.3% of net sales, a 35% increase over 1977 levels. Even at a conservatively projected 13% annual increase, illness-care costs will double between 1981 and 1989. Clearly, some action was required.

Other forces unique to Johnson & Johnson were at work. Health care is our primary business. If the preliminary scientific evidence linking life-style and health was correct, then Johnson & Johnson had a responsibility to assume industry leadership and demonstrate the feasibility of improving health through life-style change. Moreover, Johnson & Johnson management is guided by responsibilities outlined in the company's credo, which, in part, requires management to be "responsible to our employees." Management sentiment was perhaps best captured by James E. Burke, chairman and chief executive officer of Johnson & Johnson, who said that "it would be illogical for a health care company not to have healthy employees."

In combination, the forces of (1) scientific consensus linking life-styles with health, (2) financial pressure to control illness-care costs, and (3) the desire to exercise health care leadership presented Johnson & Johnson senior management with a unique opportunity to act. The *Live for Life* program was the consequence. Its original mandate in 1978 was to provide in a cost-effective manner the opportunity for Johnson & Johnson employees to become among the healthiest employees in the world. The *Live for Life* program has evolved considerably from its inception, and its current mission is to provide the direction and resources to Johnson & Johnson employees, their families, and the community that will result in healthier life-styles and help contain illness-care costs. This chapter will concentrate on how business marketing expertise was applied to the myriad obstacles confronting this effort.

MARKET ANALYSIS

Market analysis consisted of gathering as much information as possible about products, services, and procedures that were available to improve life-styles. In-depth interviews were conducted with leading experts in the field of life-style change. Site visits were arranged with projects like the *Stanford Heart Disease Prevention Program* where large-scale life-style interventions had been attempted. Existing data on life-style change programs were collected and thoroughly reviewed. By 1977, several corporations had developed employee fitness programs, and these too were analyzed. Together, the initial 6-month market analysis effort yielded one clear conclusion: the *Live for Life* program represented essentially a new venture in uncharted waters. Although some guidelines were available, the market analysis identified a number of obstacles that stood in the way of improving employee health in a cost-effective manner.

One obstacle was scientific. The science of life-style improvement was in its infancy. A clear technology did not exist to achieve precise and predictable life-style improvements among large numbers of people. Although the Stanford Three Community Study and a similar project in North Karelia, Finland suggested that life-style improvements were possible, neither supplied much insight into how to organize and implement a cost-effective effort within the work setting. Yet, such a technology would have to be developed if the *Live for Life* program was to achieve its goals of having healthier employees and cost-effectiveness. Moreover, within the behavioral science community, only limited consensus could be found on the most efficacious ways to influence life-styles. To complicate matters more, there was only questionable evidence that life-style improvements, once accomplished, could be sustained as permanent fixtures of a person's life. The specter loomed large of a high financial investment yielding at best only temporary life-style change.

In the biomedical community, even less consensus existed on the precise long-term impact of life-style improvements on illness-care costs. Although most members of the biomedical community felt health and life-styles were linked, few were willing to rank which life-style improvements would yield the highest economic dividends or specify what economic benefits could be expected from a specific life-style change. For example, the economic benefit of converting a smoker to a non-smoker or a physically unfit person to a higher level of fitness could not be calculated with existing data. Thus, the *Live for Life* program had to be launched in an atmosphere in which the economic benefits were an article of faith rather than an empirically sound rationale for action.

In many respects, the scientific obstacles confronting the *Live for Life* program paled in comparison with obstacles endemic to the business environment itself. Although some of these obstacles were specific to Johnson & Johnson, most are found within any business organization. Johnson & Johnson follows a business philosophy of decentralized decision making. Rather than one vertically structured corporation, Johnson & Johnson is composed of a large number of companies, each operating in an autonomous and independent fashion. Thus, each company's management board would have the complete say about whether to offer the *Live for Life* program to their employees. Within a decentralized business environment, a corporate decision to improve the health of all employees had to accept the reality that each autonomous company would make the final decision. In essence, the *Live for Life* program had the responsibility for improving employee life-styles in a cost-effective way but no authority to make it happen. The net consequence of a decentralized operating environment was the need to develop a *Live for Life* program that was flexible enough to accommodate the unique characteristics of a particular company while maintaining the essential core elements necessary to achieve significant life-style improvements.

Another organizational obstacle was designing a cost-effective program that could be delivered to 35,000 employees at more than 75 locations in the United States. The sheer magnitude of this task made it impossible to implement a program that relied on intensive professional intervention, which, at that time, was the most prevalent model for delivering health care services. The enormous cost of recruiting, training, and maintaining a cadre of full-time health professionals would be prohibitive. Another approach must be found.

Perhaps the most formidable obstacle was how to implement a health promotion program within what is essentially a hostile environment. Business organizations in particular are economically driven. All efforts are directed toward preserving and enhancing the economic viability of the enterprise. Programs and activities that are not seen as inherently compatible with the basic operational objectives are not well tolerated. When the *Live for Life* program was originally started, it had no evidence that it could in fact improve employee health, much less any evidence that it would enhance the economic goals of a company. Moreover, because the *Live for Life* program sought widespread employee involvement and participation, it was perceived as competing for such valuable and scarce resources as money and management and employee time. Funding and attention for the *Live for Life* program necessarily meant that other projects might not be funded or receive proper attention. Consequently, the *Live for Life* program had to minimize potential sources of hostility while competing fiercely for the limited organizational resources necessary for its success.

Another potential obstacle was the implied psychological threat felt by some people by the very nature of the *Live for Life* program. Consider the senior manager who is overweight and smokes. He is now confronted by a company program that suggests that his life-style is not optimal. Very likely this is a person who has successfully climbed the ranks over the years and has arrived at his current position only to find the rules of success and acceptance being changed. Thin is "in" and people are beginning to display no smoking signs. Such a confrontation in values can be very threatening. If so, the most straightforward way to handle this threat is to sabotage the program and do so quickly.

A related problem in any large organization is a phenomenon called *fence sitting*. Whenever any new venture (like the *Live for Life* program) is initiated, the well-honed competitive instincts in many people encourage them to sit on the fence and wait and see how the venture fares. This is a serious problem because the credibility and survival of a new venture is intimately linked to how many people accept it. Many people do not want to risk being associated with a failure. They perceive a considerable risk in jumping on the bandwagon early and publicly supporting a program before success is certain. Fence sitting is not a hostile act, but the net effect is often the same when a new venture like the *Live for Life* program is greeted by a deafening silence. Consequently, the *Live for Life* program had to be positioned in a way that minimized psychological threat and gave the appearance of a "sure bet."

A third major obstacle was the unique nature of the task itself. Ninety percent of all Johnson & Johnson employees are healthy by conventional standards. They do not have physical or psychological symptoms of illness or disease that require traditional medical interventions. In essence, they feel fine and perceive little need to change life-style activities that are often rich with immediate positive consequences, such as the satisfaction of food or the tension release of a cigarette. Of course, the *Live for Life* program could offer vague assurances of a few extra years of life, but that would be in 20 or 30 years. The argument to delay immediate gratification in return for a slightly longer life is simply not convincing. The *Live for Life* program had to do better if it was to effect a significant improvement in employee life-styles.

In summary, to be successful, the *Live for Life* program had to address and resolve myriad obstacles. Scientific consensus on how to change life-styles in an industrial environment required development, as did the technology for achieving such changes. In the absence of firm evidence, justification for scarce financial resources was needed to convince business management that the risk of the *Live for Life* program was worth the gamble. The *Live for Life* program had to be designed in ways that minimized a number of thorny obstacles endemic to any large organization. Finally, the *Live for Life* program had to gain the attention, acceptance, and sustained commitment for life-style improvement among Johnson & Johnson employees in an atmosphere where few perceived any urgent need for such changes.

DEVELOPING THE PROGRAM

The *Live for Life* program was launched like most new business ventures. A vice-president on the corporate staff with extensive experience in marketing, sales, and new business development was assigned responsibility for translating into reality the mandate to improve significantly employee life-styles in a cost-effective manner. Most new business ventures have very little time to establish their viability. *Live for Life* was not an exception. Consequently, the operational strategy was to move forward rapidly in program development, addressing and trying to resolve many obstacles simultaneously.

Technology Consensus

The *Live for Life* program required immediate direction in terms of focus and technique; namely, what life-styles should be promoted and how to do so effectively within an industrial environment. To achieve a workable consensus on program focus and technique, the management of the *Live for Life* program organized a series of round table discussions with leading experts in the behavioral sciences and biomedical communities. Each round table was given the charge to provide *Live for Life* program management with consensus advice on how best to proceed. Round tables were organized in key areas like state-of-the-art behavioral interventions, stress management, exercise, and nutrition/weight control. For 1–2 days, round table members and *Live for Life* program management engaged in freewheeling discussions on the topic at hand. Aside from keeping the discussion to a specific area, like exercise or stress management, very few constraints were placed on the participants. A chairperson was selected beforehand, whose main responsibility was to help *Live for Life* program management identify round table participants and to keep discussions generally within bounds during the meeting.

This round table approach to technology consensus had two principal advantages. Management staff members of the *Live for Life* program were afforded the opportunity to explore important state-of-the-art life-style and methodology issues in considerable detail with a panel of leading experts. Learning for management was condensed and concentrated, thus accelerating the program development process. Another advantage was the opportunity for *Live for Life* management to become personally acquainted with a cadre of leading experts in their respective fields and to introduce them to the goals and objectives of *Live for Life.* Such contact would prove invaluable later when *Live for Life* management needed to turn to these experts for assistance in the development of specific health promotion programs (e.g., weight control, smoking cessation).

A consistent picture began to emerge from this series of round tables. The primary life-style factors that the *Live for Life* program should address included weight, nutrition, exercise, stress, smoking, and alcohol use. In order to achieve sustained life-style improvements, the *Live for Life* program must simultaneously provide (1) opportunities for employees to learn the skills required for life-style improvement, and (2) an environment at work that supported and encouraged individual life-style improvements. Consensus was reached that health behavior is a function of a reciprocal interaction between individuals and their environment. To the extent possible, individual decisions to make a life-style improvement should be promoted through the convenient availability of effective programs at the worksite, a consumer benefit, coupled with changes in the work environment that supported the life-style improvement. For example, an effort to encourage reductions in excess weight should combine a convenient and effective weight control program at the worksite with a concerted effort to promote the purchase of lower calorie foods in the company cafeteria and vending machines. It made little sense to encourage positive life-styles without concurrent alterations in the work environment that helped produce or sustain negative life-styles in the first place. In essence, the work environment is a very effective channel for the distribution of health promotion services. A technology for sustained life-style improvement must address individuals and their environment.

Consensus was especially strong on the pivotal role of the social environment. It was seen as potentially the single most powerful factor the *Live for Life* program could influence in support of positive life-styles. High employee participation was a key factor that was very much under the control of the *Live for Life* program. To the extent that the *Live for Life* program attracted large numbers of employees in such programs as exercise, smoking cessation, stress management, and weight control, a healthier social environment would be created. High participation in the *Live for Life* program would be a catalyst. It would provide critical support for sustained life-style improvement among program participants as well as acting as a magnet to draw more employees into health enhancement activities.

In summary, the key strategy in effective life-style improvement technology became the creation and implementation of a health promotion program that would achieve the most visible and widespread employee participation possible. The *Live for Life* program was not aimed at individuals at high risk. It was a program that strategically sought and depended upon the attention and visible participation of the majority of Johnson & Johnson employees.

A Process, Not a Program

It was very difficult to conceptualize any program or series of programs that would suitably attract the sustained interest and involvement of a majority of employees. Given the primary strategy of high participation, the *Live for Life* program could not be marketed successfully as a simple collection of health promotion programs such as exercise and weight control. Product identification was weak. No structure existed for holding these programs together. Instead, the *Live for Life* program had to be conceptualized as a process that systematically built high employee participation over time. The process became the structural source of continuity or glue that held essential components of the *Live for Life* program together. Consequently, the *Live for Life* program was constructed as a total health enhancement system that consisted of multiple components. There are a number of important advantages to designing and marketing a health promotion process rather than a program. New components can be added over time, and old or ineffective components can be replaced while the basic system remains intact. Moreover, a process is far more flexible and responsive to the unique health enhancement needs and desires of a diverse set of employees and companies than the mere collection of rigid program offerings. This advantage was especially important, considering the goal of fostering high participation and the need to market the *Live for Life* program to a group of very autonomous and decentralized companies. Perhaps most important is the market control afforded by a system. When a company purchases a system, the system supplier has far more leverage to control what component parts or services are used in that system over time. By analogy, IBM markets computer *systems*. Once the system is in place, the purchaser is far more likely to return to IBM for replacement parts and new features. In a similar vein, the *Live for Life* program is a health enhancement system.

Conceptualized as a process, the *Live for Life* program development activity concentrated on identifying, testing, and refining the initial collection of component parts that were essential to make the system operate. Considerable attention was devoted to how the component parts should be organized or positioned in order to achieve the maximum participation possible.

In Search of a McDonald's Hamburger

The *Live for Life* program is a process. It is also a service. Marketing a service successfully requires a standardized operational system that produces the same level of quality and performance whenever and wherever that service is delivered. A textbook example is McDonald's hamburgers. Whether it is Hong Kong, The Bronx, or Davenport, Iowa, McDonald's offers a predictable and consistent level of service in terms of products, atmosphere, convenience, and even restrooms. The *Live for Life* program management sought a similar operational system or process that delivered predictable and consistent health enhancement performance and quality whenever and wherever the *Live for Life* program was offered. Several steps were taken to achieve this end.

A common unifying theme was needed to link all *Live for Life* products and services. The title of the program itself, *Life for Life,* was selected for this specific purpose. All health enhancement activities could be promoted under the same rubric of *Live for Life.* A rainbow logo was established, thus allowing all products and services associated with the *Live for Life* program to be easily recognized. For example, all *Live for Life* program materials such as weight control manuals and smoking cessation manuals were bound in the same colorful binders with the *Live for Life* program logo prominently displayed. At a minimum, a uniform packaging and logo use policy ensured that all *Live for Life* program products and services would have the same high-quality appearance wherever they appeared.

To achieve predictable, uniform results, all *Live for Life* programs must contain the same basic set of products and services. Because the *Live for Life* program was originally conceived as a comprehensive health promotion program, a concept of *core Live for Life* program components emerged. The core components took shape around those services that were considered absolutely essential to the process of achieving high employee participation. These core services included (1) a health screen that informed participants of their current health status; (2) a life-style seminar that introduced participants to health promotion programs available through the *Live for Life* program; (3) focused health promotion programs in nutrition, weight control, smoking cessation, stress management, and exercise; (4) consulting expertise in the design and maintenance of a healthy work environment; and (5) programs and activities that sustained participation over time.

The core components concept strengthened the marketing flexibility of the *Live for Life* program. On the one hand, it retained the ability of the *Live for Life* program to have the essential elements of the process at work in any company location. On the other hand, individual companies could add to the process those unique elements that characterized their company needs and desires. An example is exercise facilities. The *Live for Life* program recommends the convenient availability to lockers, showers, and some exercise space. How a company responds to this recommendation depends on many factors, including available space, access to community facilities, and so on. Although a company may decide to build an exercise facility on site, the *Live for Life* program does not require (or necessarily support) such a capital expenditure. In short, the decision to offer employees a convenient set of exercise programs is not an option with the *Live for Life* program, but the exact details of how, when, and where such programs are offered is very much a company decision.

Identifying the Customer

At first glance, the real customers of the *Live for Life* program are Johnson & Johnson employees. They are the target audience whose participation and allegiance is sought. *Live for Life* programs and services are designed to meet their health enhancement needs. Moreover, containing the illness-care costs of Johnson & Johnson employees is the ultimate challenge and goal of the *Live for Life* program. There is no doubt that Johnson & Johnson employees are primary customers because it is their actions over time that will decide the fate of the *Live for Life* program. The only problem is that, as customers, employees do not pay for the program. A company's management does.

A company's management is the other primary customer for the *Live for Life* program and for very good reasons. Ideas do not survive in a business environment without top management support. The *Live for Life* program is no exception. Consequently, the *Live for Life* program is positioned to top management of the various Johnson & Johnson companies as a package that will immediately provide a substantial employee benefit and, over time, give management some leverage to control illness-care costs.

As the purchaser of the *Live for Life* program, company management becomes part of a customer base whose needs and desires must be satisfied as well. One obvious need is a program that is demonstratively attractive to employees. The employee benefit aspect of the *Live for Life* program must be clear, immediate, and recognizable. Equally important, however, the program cannot be seen as disruptive to the basic operational environment. Business must come first! The *Live for Life* program must enhance the business process, not interfere with the basic organizational objectives. Moreover, the program must reflect the management and operational style of a particular company. Finally, the program must be accountable to management for results. Every year proposed *Live for Life* program funding will receive the same intense scrutiny from management as any other aspect of the business. Over time, the *Live for Life* program will receive management resources commensurate with its demonstrable contribution to the overall goals and objectives of the business organization.

Operational Philosophy

The *Live for Life* program's success hinges on its ability to sell healthier life-styles to large numbers of Johnson & Johnson employees. Although the program is evolving a technology for selling health, the process is guided by several philosophical assumptions that accentuate consumer benefits. The process must present a positive approach to health. Employees are more likely to participate in programs that are positive and upbeat in style and content. This is especially true because participation is voluntary and on the employees' own time. Thus, *Live for Life* programs must compete for the attention, time, and sustained interest of employees in an environment where the alternatives—lunch with friends, shopping, TV, time with family—are powerful and very appealing. Potential participants will be attracted by an approach that emphasizes the immediate benefits of the program, for example, better relationships, more energy, greater productivity. They will be repelled by a negative approach, for example, an emphasis on cancer, heart disease, and early death. Moreover, the initial experiences of employees with *Live for Life* programs must be positive if they are to remain actively involved in the program. Not only must the program style and content be positive, but the information and experience derived from participation must lead to positive benefits for employees. Weight control programs must produce desirable weight losses. Smoking cessation programs must help employees stop smoking. Stress management programs must equip employees with beneficial skills to reduce unwanted effects of stress. Exercise programs must lead to an enhanced sense of fitness and well-being.

The process must be oriented toward healthy people. Ninety percent of all Johnson & Johnson employees are healthy by conventional standards, and they represent the market for the *Live for Life* program. They do not have physical or psychological symptoms of illness or disease that require medical intervention. *Live for Life* programs are designed for employees who feel healthy. They want to improve or enhance those life-style characteristics that are directly linked to long-term health and a high quality of life. They are successful people who have many strengths. They see *Live for Life* program participation as a unique opportunity to improve and further enhance their existing strengths.

Live for Life programs are not designed for those few employees who, at a given point in time, need professional or medical assistance. The company medical department and employee assistance programs are available for employees needing such assistance. *Live for Life* program leaders must view participants as healthy. *Live for Life* programs are not therapy and should never be conducted as such. A program leader's attitude should always reflect the reality that participants are there voluntarily to improve their health. They are not there to receive some professional treatment for problems.

The process must emphasize the practical. Participants in *Live for Life* programs expect to learn how to do things. How to lose weight, how to stop smoking, how to manage stress, and how to start an exercise program are the kinds of questions to which participants want answers. The *Live for Life* program is an opportunity to improve health. Consequently, employees want to leave *Live for Life* programs with practical suggestions and guidelines for actually improving some aspect of their life-styles that will result in improved health. The accent is on *action*. Program leaders must create an environment in which information and skills are delivered to participants in a way that leads to direct application and utility in their daily lives. By definition, practical information is that which may be easily incorporated and used by individuals with modern life-styles.

Organization and Leadership

Responsibility for managing a *Live for Life* program resides with the company management that purchases the program. This decision on ownership is consistent with the decentralized operating philosophy of Johnson & Johnson. More important, it strategically positions responsibility for program success squarely where, in reality, it belongs: with company management. As soon as the program is purchased, it is no longer the Johnson & Johnson Corporate *Live for Life* program. It is the Personal Products *Live for Life* program, the Ethicon *Live for Life* program, the McNeil Consumer Products *Live for Life* program, and so on. Of course, an important component of the *Live for Life* service's being purchased is consulting expertise on the organization and operation of a *Live for Life* program. But final program decisions are placed in the hands of a company's management. It is *their Live for Life* program.

The basic structure of company *Live for Life* programs is that of a volunteer organization headed by a person or persons selected by top management because of their managerial abilities. It is this initial selection of managers (normally called co-chairpersons) that represents the single most important aspect of organizational structuring. These co-chairpersons serve as the keystone of the *Live for Life* program organization on the sites, and like the keystones of ancient Roman architecture, they are held in place by pressure from both sides; on the one side, top management, and on the other, those persons to whom the majority of the benefits for the program accrue. It is this dual pressure that represents both the strength and problems of this particular position. Normally the managers selected as co-chairpersons come from key operational areas such as manufacturing, marketing, or research. A cross-section of persons is desirable so that not only will major departments be represented but also so that those persons selected will have some knowledge of the talented persons in each of the various areas. It is then up to the co-chairperson to recruit selectively from the volunteers that come forward when the program is introduced. Once the volunteers are selected, they work with the *Live for Life* program corporate staff through a position known as *program coordinator* to put into effect the programs referred to earlier. Training, motivation, and a firm knowledge of the company's primary business are important criteria when selecting a program coordinator. The key to working with volunteers is to provide them with immediate gratification and easily identifiable objectives. No vague promises, no poorly defined goals will maintain volunteer leadership over time. Because all of those involved will have other things to do with their time (indeed, they will have managers more than happy to assist them in identifying those things), it is important that the volunteers all feel responsible for a specific part of the program and its implementation. Once such assignments are given and clear objectives are set, then the program can continue. It is hard to underestimate the importance of these goal-setting activities and constant positive feedback. Volunteer leadership seems to work best when given a limited tenure. Experience has shown that 1-year terms of duty seem to be preferred. Furthermore, when replacing volunteer leadership, care should be given not to fall into the habit of replacing senior managers with middle managers, middle managers with supervisors, and so on. The quality and status of the position can only be maintained over time if managers of the same corporate level replace the initial leadership cadre.

This volunteer structure offers a number of advantages. One is economic. The financial outlays necessary to manage a *Live for Life* program are measurably less if this responsibility is placed with existing employees. The process of delivering *Live for Life* to 35,000 employees in a cost-effective way becomes more feasible when the 35,000 employees are viewed as a potential source of volunteer leaders as opposed to simply consumers of *Live for Life* program services.

Another advantage is the ability to identify and tap an extremely talented group of people who have already demonstrated a capacity to get things done within the business organization. Senior members of this volunteer leadership cadre are recruited from middle- to upper-management ranks. These are people who know the organization well and have management experience. This expertise is especially important because, in essence, a *Live for Life* program is established as a business entity within a company's larger business framework. It has a budget, objectives, and decision-making authority to plan and execute the necessary steps to achieve these objectives. The senior group of volunteer leaders functions much like a company management board and, indeed, is responsible to the company's management for program success.

A third advantage is the immediate creation of a core group of employees dedicated to the success of their *Live for Life* program. This group, combined with the 10% to 20% of any employee population already firmly committed to health enhancement activities, forms the nucleus of a critical mass often necessary to launch a *Live for Life* program.

Finally, the employees of a company are often in the best positions to know the health enhancement needs and interests of their fellow employees. They can receive feedback directly and frequently on program quality, performance, and direction. Such information is invaluable in delivering a service such as the *Live for Life* program.

The disadvantages of a volunteer leadership system primarily relate to the time constraints and business priorities of the volunteers' own jobs. The *Live for Life* program necessarily comes second. Despite this major drawback, a volunteer leadership system can work quite well if the proper people are recruited and management support is clear and unequivocal.

PROGRAM OPERATION

Live for Life Corporate Staff

Responsibility for coordinating and delivering *Live for Life* programs to the family of Johnson & Johnson companies rests with the *Live for Life* program corporate staff. This small group provides the technical assistance and support to a company as it builds its own *Live for Life* program. Its primary expertise resides in supplying participating companies with the consulting expertise, training, core program components, professional services, and promotional materials necessary for program success. *Live for Life* program staff are also responsible for program development and evaluation.

A program coordinator from the *Live for Life* staff is assigned to each participating company. The program coordinator functions as an account executive and is the essential link between the company and the full range of *Live for Life* program services available through the *Live for Life* program corporate staff. The program coordinator is absolutely critical to program success. Although the program coordinator has no authority or responsibility over the day-to-day operations of a company's *Live for Life* program, skillful consultation and salesmanship with company leadership and management work to ensure that the *Live for Life* program process is properly planned, organized, and implemented in a way that satisfies the health enhancement needs of the entire customer base.

Sales Presentation to Company Management

The *Live for Life* program process begins with a sales presentation to a company's management board. When the *Live for Life* program was in its early development phase, this presentation concentrated primarily upon the company's illness-care cost history. This particular sales technique always got the management board's attention because it was not difficult to paint a picture of rapidly accelerating illness-care costs. The *Live for Life* program was positioned as a potential mechanism to help control illness-care costs and, in the process, to provide employees with a substantial employee benefit.

Now that the *Live for Life* program has been operating at many Johnson & Johnson companies for some time, the sales presentation has become easier. Management board members no longer have to make a decision to offer their employees the *Live for Life* program on faith alone. They can and do send a task force to companies with ongoing *Live for Life* programs and examine the process firsthand. Moreover, considerable evidence is accumulating on the *Live for Life* program's impact on employees' health, life-styles, and attitudes. In combination, the potential for economic saving, the success of the *Live for Life* program at other companies, and the documented impact of the program on employees makes the *Live for Life* program an extremely attractive investment.

The management board is asked to make three commitments: to give financial resources, management time, and responsiveness to employee requests for environmental improvements. Finding sufficient financial resources is often the easiest commitment to fulfill. Management time is a much more scarce resource. Yet, management board members are made aware that the success of their *Live for Life* program is linked to their willingness to recruit talented middle- to upper-management people to serve as senior volunteer leaders. By definition, good senior leaders must be the kind of people who currently are contributing 50 hr per week or more to the company's success. The management board must be willing to allow these people to give only 35–40 hr per week to their jobs; the remaining time is devoted to managing the *Live for Life* program.

Finally, the volunteer leadership group is charged with the responsibility to recommend to the management board a range of significant environmental improvements that the leadership feels are necessary to encourage and support widespread employee participation and life-style change. The management board must be responsive to these requests and be willing to take those steps that, in their business judgment, are appropriate and sound. Development of exercise facilities, a company smoking policy, and "flextime" are examples of proposed environmental improvements to which management boards are often asked to respond.

Selection of Volunteer Leaders

A management board member is typically assigned operational responsibility for the *Live for Life* program. This person is often the vice-president of personnel, but in a number of companies the vice-president of finance is selected. The first task is to identify and recruit the senior group of volunteer leaders. Originally, the *Live for Life* program recommended a grass roots approach in which all employees interested in helping to lead the company's *Live for Life* program were asked to come forward. About 15% to 20% of the employees of a site volunteered, and an elaborate interviewing process was conducted to identify among the volunteers those 5–10 people who should comprise the senior leadership group. The advantage of this approach was the instant formation of a core group of employees throughout the company committed to the success of the *Live for Life* program. The disadvantages were considerable, however, and they included a tremendous amount of interviewing time and the inherent inefficiencies associated with trying to organize this large group of volunteers into task forces and assigning them meaningful tasks. Confusion, rather than purposeful action, was the norm.

The *Live for Life* program now recommends more of a top-down approach to leadership selection. The management board representative selects the top two or three senior managers (*Live for Life* program co-chairpersons). The co-chairpersons in turn select five to seven managers to lead task forces organized around such key areas as exercise, smoking cessation, stress management, weight control/nutrition, publicity, and general health knowledge. The task force leaders, in turn, recruit a cross-section of employees as task force members.

Working closely with a *Live for Life* program coordinator, the volunteer leadership members assume primary responsibility for the following management and administrative functions:

1. Develop and submit to management yearly program plans, participation objectives, and budget requirements
2. Recommend environmental improvements to the management board
3. Develop, execute, and manage a strategy for achieving program plans and participation targets
4. Evaluate the need for a permanent employee or employees to administer the programs following the initial start-up phase
5. Request health enhancement services and materials from the *Live for Life* program corporate staff and other vendors as required
6. Prepare periodic reports to management on program results, including participation achievements and employee health and life-style improvements

Health Screen

For most employees, the process begins with participation in the *Live for Life* program health screen. The health screen is promoted as a unique opportunity for all employees to find out how healthy they are and to learn much about health in the process. The health screen is offered on company time and takes about 1 hr to complete. All employees who wish to participate in *Live for Life* exercise programs must complete the health screen. Health and life-style variables collected and analyzed during the health screen include biometric (e.g., blood lipids, blood pressure, body fat, height and weight, and estimated maximal oxygen uptake), behavioral (e.g., smoking, alcohol use, physical activity, dental hygiene practices, nutrition practices, coronary-prone behavior pattern, stress management skill use, sleep quality, human relations, and human potential), and attitudinal measures (e.g., general well-being, satisfaction with working conditions, relations with others, growth opportunities, ability to handle job strain, job involvement, job self-esteem, and organizational commitment).

The *Live for Life* program corporate staff is responsible for providing the health screen service. The company leaders are primarily responsible for the organization, promotion, recruitment, and scheduling of employees into the health screen, although the *Live for Life* program corporate staff members are available to provide extensive advice and logistical assistance. An 80% participation rate is the recommended target.

Life-Style Seminar

The *Live for Life* program process continues with a life-style seminar that is usually scheduled about 6 weeks after an employee completes the health screen. The life-style seminar is the primary vehicle for introducing employees to their company's *Live for Life* program. Personal responsibility for health is emphasized, especially within the context of a *Live for Life* program in which the company has committed itself to creating a work environment rich in opportunities to improve and maintain personal health. Employee health screen results are returned at this point via an attractive document called a *life-style profile.* The life-style profile is positioned as a way to determine "how healthy you are," and provides the basis for taking action to improve health through *Live for Life* program participation. Upcoming *Live for Life* program health enhancement opportunities are reviewed and promoted. The life-style seminar is offered on company time to groups of about 50 employees each, and takes about 3 hr.

Live for Life program corporate staff are responsible for conducting the life-style seminar and ensuring that each employee who participated in the health screen receives his or her life-style profile at this point. Company leaders are primarily responsible for the promotion, recruitment, and scheduling of employees into the life-style seminar. They are also responsible for presenting to employees the health enhancement opportunities available through their company's *Live for Life* program during the coming year. A 70% employee participation target is recommended.

Life-Style Improvement Programs

An essential component of the *Live for Life* program process is the ongoing opportunity for employees to improve or maintain their health through participation in exercise, weight control, nutrition, smoking cessation, and stress management programs. The employees' participation is voluntary and is done on their own time. *Live for Life* program corporate staff members have developed the set of core action programs described in Table 1.

In addition to action programs, *Live for Life* program corporate staff have developed a range of shorter educational and promotional programs built around such themes as breast self-examination, biofeedback, nutrition, blood pressure, and carbon monoxide analysis for smokers.

Live for Life program corporate staff are responsible for making available to participating companies this set of carefully tested and evaluated programs as well as trained professional leaders to conduct the programs. Moreover, *Live for Life* program corporate staff conduct ongoing audits to ensure that all life-style improvement programs meet established quality and performance standards. A report on the quality and performance of all life-style improvement programs supplied by *Live for Life* program corporate staff is issued to company leaders on a regular basis.

Company leaders are responsible for the ongoing selection, promotion, recruitment, and scheduling of employees into life-style improvement programs in the core areas of exercise, weight control/nutrition, smoking cessation, and stress management. They need not select programs available through *Live for Life* program corporate staff. The strategy is to offer a combination of life-style improvement programs that achieve high employee participation and, as a consequence, fundamentally

Table 1. Descriptions of the Live for Life *Program Core Action Programs*

Action program	Description
Smoking cessation	A 9-session program that teaches employees how to kick the habit.
Weight control	A 10-session program that emphasizes eating fewer calories and burning up more through regular exercise.
Exercise	A series of 12-week aerobic exercise groups.
Applied stress management	An 8-session program designed to teach basic mental and physical relaxation skills.
Yoga	A 12-session program that introduces employees to basic yoga exercises and skills.
Personal power	A 10-session program to teach employees how to manage stres through improved personal assertiveness.
Nutrition	An 8-session program designed to cover the essential aspect prudent eating pattern.

restructure the social environment at work. In consultation with the program coordinator, company leaders are encouraged to establish participation targets in the core program areas. Although these participation targets will vary from company to company, depending upon differences in employee health status, representative participation targets during the first year are as follows:

Participation targets	Percentage of eligible employees
Weight control	25% of all overweight employees
Smoking cessation	20% of all employees who smoke
Stress management	20% of all employees
Exercise	40% of all employees

Programs To Sustain Participation

The introduction of a novel health enhancement program like the *Live for Life* program invariably creates widespread employee interest and involvement. The challenge is to sustain high program participation after the novelty wears off and initial enthusiasm subsides. Company leaders in consultation with the program coordinator must begin planning ways to sustain participation during the early phases of program development and execution. One program often considered is an incentive system. In business, regular feedback to employees on their performance has been shown time and again to be a critical aspect of sustaining and improving performance over time. This basic management principle also applies to health. Employees participate in life-style improvement programs to the extent that they perceive positive consequences (feedback) for doing so. Many employees find a structured incentive system to be a powerful source of positive consequences. Participating in various *Live for Life* program activities can earn points, and incentives can be awarded to those employees who earn a predetermined number of points.

The *Live for Life* program corporate staff offers participating companies the basic structure for an incentive system called the *life-style scorecard.* On a quarterly basis, employees receive a complete summary of all life-style points earned for participating in a wide array of *Live for Life* program activities, including fitness, health screens, life-style seminar, and other life-style improvement programs. Company leaders may use the life-style scorecard system or develop their own mechanism for a structured incentive system.

Regular feedback to company leaders and management on program perfor-ance is also a necessary feature to sustain participation. Company leaders are more husiastic and committed to program promotion when they receive regular feed- on their success to date. Positive consequences for leaders are directly linked to evidence that their volunteer efforts are paying off. In the short run, regular reports of program participation and results, such as the number of employees attending weight control programs and the average weight loss, provide essential feedback. Over time, a concise summary of overall program impact on employee health and life-styles is a richly satisfying reward for leaders. *Live for Life* program corporate staff are responsible for supplying regular feedback reports to company leaders and their management.

Sustained program participation is also enhanced by providing health screen opportunities on a regular basis. *Live for Life* program corporate staff recommend a health screen every 2 years. During second and subsequent health screens, employees can see quantitative improvements in their health and life-styles as a consequence of *Live for Life* program participation.

Another method to sustain program involvement is regular follow-up with participants. *Live for Life* program corporate staff members have developed a system in which all employees who participated in life-style improvement programs are contacted by phone or mail at regular intervals after the completion of that program. The primary purpose is to provide participants with a minimum structure through which they can report progress in sustaining life-style improvements (e.g., weight loss, smoking cessation, regular exercise) that were initially achieved during the structured action program. The follow-up system also serves to reinforce the key life-style activities considered essential to sustained life-style improvement (e.g., regular weighing and counting calories in weight control, regular practice of stress management skills). Moreover, regular follow-up provides program management with valuable information on effectiveness over time.

Of equal importance to sustained life-style improvements is the need to establish a mechanism for replacing company leaders. Company leadership assignments should last no longer than 1 year and may indeed be less. Plans should be developed early for the orderly transfer of management responsibility from one set of leaders to another. Part of this process may involve hiring permanent personnel to assume many of the daily administrative duties of the *Live for Life* program following the introductory phase. This person(s) may direct fitness activities as well as coordinate other *Live for Life* program activities. A permanent person assigned *Live for Life* program responsibilities, either full or part time, adds much-needed continuity to the program over time.

Creating a Healthy Environment

The primary responsibility of company leaders is to create a work environment that supports and encourages positive health practices among the greatest number of employees possible. Offering regular, convenient, and attractive life-style-improvement programs will go a long way toward creating a positive social environment based on high employee participation. Other aspects of the work environment are targets for improvement as well. Examples of several possible environmental improvements in key health and life-style areas include:

Fitness
- shower and locker facilities on site
- exercise facilities either on site or rented from local organizations

Weight Control/Nutrition
- scales in restrooms
- availability of convenient nutrition information where food is sold
- availability of nutritious foods in the company cafeteria and vending machines

Stress Management
- employee assistance program to provide professional treatment and referral services to troubled employees
- availability of management training programs designed to improve boss–subordinate relations
- flextime
- carpooling
- self-administered blood pressure equipment

Smoking Cessation
- smoking policy
- availability of *Live for Life* program thank-you-for-not-smoking signs

Publicity
- *Live for Life* program newsletter
- *Live for Life* program bulletin board and information display area
- comprehensive recruitment brochure
- health fairs
- poster displays for upcoming programs

RESULTS AND IMPLICATIONS

Better employee health should ultimately result in a significant reduction in premature morbidity and mortality, especially in health problems attributable to unhealthy behaviors and life-styles that are amenable to modification in the worksetting. However, the success of the *Live for Life* program in achieving this goal cannot be measured directly within a short time period. To do so would require far more employees and resources than are available. Consequently, in September 1979, a 2-year epidemiological evaluation was initiated to assess the degree to which the *Live for Life* program achieved significant and sustained improvements in those employee health and life-style characteristics that are likely to result in long-term good health.

Simultaneously, efforts were undertaken to monitor the degree of employee participation in the *Live for Life* program and to develop mechanisms for assessing the potential economic impact on the corporation of improved employee health. Three employee measurement systems have evolved: health and life-style improvement, program participation, and economic costs and benefits. These measurement systems are unique in industry and offer an exciting opportunity to evaluate and document how well the *Live for Life* program achieves its original goals.

Epidemiological Evaluation

Design

Ideally, a randomized prospective controlled trial of the *Live for Life* program would be the most convincing test of the intervention. For a number of reasons, this design was not possible. When using an educational campaign and facilities for life-style improvement over an entire site or factory, one cannot keep individuals randomly assigned to a control group from being exposed to the intervention. Random assignment of company sites also proved impossible.

Instead, a quasi-experimental research strategy was considered feasible and very suitable for evaluation purposes. Designs of this sort were described by Campbell and Stanley (1963) and further developed by Cook and Campbell (1976). The *Live for Life* program is evaluated employing what Campbell and Stanley term a non-equivalent control groups design, which is described next.

Treatment group	O	X	O
- - - - - - - -	- - -	- - -	- - -
Control group	O		O

The O's refer to observations or health screens and the X represents the intervention or *Live for Life* program. The hatched line indicates that the groups are not randomized. Thus, the treatment group represents four companies where the *Live for Life* program was introduced from September 1979 to May 1980. The control group contains five sites with no intervention except the health screen and the return of health and life-style information to participants.

The evaluation time period is 2 years. The design as applied to the *Live for Life* program can be schematized as follows:

Treatment group		O_1	O_2	O_3
		- - -	- - -	- - -
			X	
Control group	O_1	O_2	O_3	

The O_1, O_2, and O_3 observations or health screens occur at yearly intervals. Thus, for the treatment group the O_1 health screen occurred before the *Live for Life*

Table 2. Distribution by Sex and Type of Plant of the Initial Study Sample for the Epidemiological Evaluation of the Live for Life *Program (as of July 1, 1980)*

	Male		Female		Total	
	Treatment	Control	Treatment	Control	Treatment	Control
Screened	808	803	798	637	1,606	1,440
Not screened[a]	281	287	252	285	533	572
Total	1,089	1,090	1,050	922	2,139	2,012
Screened as % of total	74.2	73.7	76.0	69.1	75.1	71.6

[a]Preliminary estimates by use of a nonrespondent survey. Approximately 17% of the individuals selected in the nonrespondent survey were either not employed or were ineligible for the study at baseline.

program began. The O_2 health screen occurs a year into the program, and the O_3 health screen takes place at the end of the second year of the program. Similarly spaced health screens in the absence of the *Live for Life* programs are planned for the control sites.

The Population

At baseline, the treatment group consisted of approximately 2,100 employees at four Johnson & Johnson facilities and the control group consisted of approximately 2,000 employees at five additional Johnson & Johnson companies. All treatment and control groups are located in the same geographical region (central New Jersey and northeastern Pennsylvania).

As of July 1, 1980, the distribution of the initial study sample by sex and type of plant was as is shown in Table 2.

Sampling Procedures

Health and life-style measures are collected on all employees who participate in the *Live for Life* program health screen at baseline and Year 1 and Year 2. All employees at the treatment and control companies are actively encouraged to participate. The primary study focus is on the cohort of employees in the treatment and control sites who participate in the health screen at baseline and at Year 2. This cohort will steadily shrink in size over the 2-year evaluation period due to an estimated 15% employee turnover rate and an estimated 70% health screen recapture rate. Cross-sectional comparisons are also planned, especially for management use.

Employees at treatment and control sites who did not participate in the health screen were designated as *nonrespondents*. A nonrespondent sampling methodology was developed and executed by Research Triangle Institute (RTI). The purpose was to make possible comparisons across all employees in all plants and to determine if responders differed from nonresponders.

Preliminary Findings

Preliminary results on the cohort of employees attending both the baseline and Year 1 health screen (excluding one treatment company because its Year 1 health screen data are not completely collected and analyzed) are very exciting. The evidence shown in Table 3 clearly suggests that the treatment cohort, in comparison with controls, consistently shows greater improvements in the major health and life-style areas addressed by the *Live for Life* program.

In summary, the very preliminary baseline 1-year comparison available at this point strongly supports the contention that the *Live for Life* program is capable of achieving significant and meaningful improvements in the health and life-styles of Johnson & Johnson employees. The findings are consistent across the range of core programs areas. Although these preliminary results are very encouraging, full documentation of the total sustained impact of the *Live for Life* program awaits full completion of the 2-year epidemiological study in mid-1982.

Table 3. Preliminary Findings of the Epidemiological Study of the Live for Life *Program*

		% Change Baseline − 1 Year		
Health and life-style area	Health screen measure	Treatment (N = 737)	Control (N = 680)	p
Fitness	Aerobic calories/kg/week	43	6	.001
Weight control	% above ideal weight	−1	6	.001
Smoking cessation	% current smokers	−15	−4	.05
Stress management	General well-being	5	2	.001
	% with elevated blood pressure (≥ 140/90)	−32	−9	—
Employee attitudes	Self-reported sick days	−9	14	.05
	Satisfaction with working conditions	3	− 7	.001
	Satisfaction with personal relations at work	1	−3	.001
	Ability to handle job strain	0	−2	.001
	Job involvement	2	0	—
	Commitment to the organization	0	−2	—
	Job self-esteem	0	−2	.05
	Satisfaction with growth opportunities	−1	−3	—

Participation Evaluation

Live for Life program corporate staff members have developed a participation system designed to (1) provide program and company management with timely information about the frequency and quality of employee participation; (2) provide employees with motivational feedback on performance; and (3) collect comprehensive information for evaluating the impact of individual program participation on health and life-style variables as well as economic factors. The latest version of the participation system incorporates the latest technology in data entry and data base design, which minimizes data entry error rates ($< .1\%$) and maximizes system flexibility. The system, which is a modular configuration, includes the following major subsystems:

- The *employee roster subsystem* contains complete demographical information on each site employee as well as certain status indicators and summary information from other subsystems.
- The *lifestyle improvement subsystem* captures total and individual attendance data and pre-, post-, and follow-up measurements for each participant enrolled in ongoing life-style improvement programs of a specific duration.
- The *special event subsystem* collects total and, whenever possible, individual attendance data for onetime activities that require no pre-, post-, or follow-up measurements.
- The *fitness activity subsystem* tracks fitness activities of program participants and includes algorithms for calculating aerobic fitness points (based on the Cooper aerobic points system). This system has the advantage of capturing employee activities at home and the worksite.

Market Penetration

On the basis of participation system data, the four test companies in the epidemiological study achieved the following participation levels in core program areas:

Health screen	76% of all employees
Life-style seminars	65% of all employees
Life-style improvement programs	
Weight control	23% of all overweight employees
Smoking cessation	20% of all employees who smoke
Stress management	17% of all employees
Fitness	20% to 40% of all employees

Participation data strongly suggest that the *Live for Life* program process is capable of achieving high and sustained involvement among employees. At any given point in time, 40% to 60% of all employees are involved in some aspect of a *Live for Life* program. This level of participation is considered critical to overall program success.

Economic Evaluation

Objective and Rationale

The objective of the economic evaluation is to assess the degree to which the *Live for Life* program is cost-effective and offers the corporation economic benefits over time. The rationale for pursuing such an objective is straightforward. The *Live for Life* program is conducted within a business environment where competition for scarce resources such as money, management time, space, and materials is a fact of life. Some may argue that the program is a significant employee benefit and that cost justification is unimportant. On the other hand, if management can be reasonably confident that there is a potentially large economic opportunity associated with a successful program, a convincing rationale exists for management to commit itself and financial resources to the *Live for Life* program concept.

The challenge is to document the potential economic benefits of improvements in employee health. The *Live for Life* program offers an exciting opportunity to pursue this challenge. Relationships can be documented between economic variables (e.g., illness-care costs, turnover, employee attitudes) and concomitant life-style and health measures collected for the epidemiological evaluation. If economic linkages were documented, *Live for Life* program corporate staff members would be in an excellent position to produce actionable reports that would enable management to make prudent program spending decisions and provide the necessary feedback to measure economic benefits over time. The end product would be the guts for a unique human resource accounting system—a concept the accounting profession has struggled with for many years. Moreover, this would be an important adjunct to any health cost containment effort, and economic measurements (in dollars) would be consistent with those used in conventional management decision making.

Strategy

Maximization of program benefits depends upon the efficient allocation of resources to those areas that offer the greatest economic opportunity and probability of success. Although there is a proliferation of literature discussing the economic merits of various health promotion efforts, there is very little substantive information about cost justification, particularly for an employed population. Therefore, *Live for Life* program corporate staff are evaluating empirical links between specific

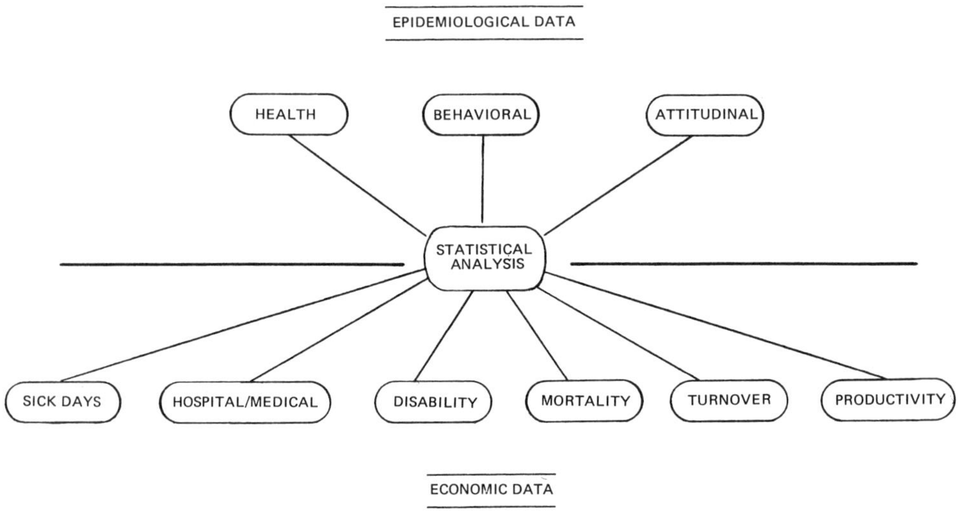

Figure 1. Facets of the program evaluation of the *Live for Life*(TM) program.

health and life-style factors collected during the health screen and internal illness-care cost data (Figure 1).

This approach bypasses the traditional effort to supply the intermediary link from health and life-style measures to disease incidence to economic assessment. For example, the economic cost of smokers will be assessed by comparing the average illness-care costs associated with smokers and nonsmokers. It will be assumed that some substantial fraction of the cost difference is the benefit recoverable by successfully encouraging a smoker to become a nonsmoker.

SUMMARY

Live for Life is in the business of selling health. It was created by Johnson & Johnson in response to the perception that a tremendous opportunity existed to improve the life quality of Johnson & Johnson employees significantly and, in the process, realize an economic benefit. Marketing expertise was systematically applied to overcome many obstacles within and outside the business environment as the program took shape and evolved over time. Consensus on a technology for improving life-styles in the workplace was achieved primarily through round table discussions with leading experts. As a product, the *Live for Life* program evolved as a process aimed at achieving high employee participation. Standardized operating procedures were developed to ensure a reliable and consistent delivery of health promotion services wherever the *Live for Life* program was offered. *Live for Life* program services had to satisfy the needs of a diverse customer base including employees and management. Because the *Live for Life* program was in the business of selling health to essentially healthy people, the marketing strategy emphasized the positive benefits consumers would experience as a consequence of participation in *Live for Life* program activities. The *Live for Life* program process begins with its acceptance and support by top management. Volunteer employee leaders are recruited to manage a company's program. Employees begin the process by participating in a health screen, and results are returned in the context of a life-style seminar. A series of core life-style improvement programs are offered in areas such as smoking cessation, weight control, nutrition, fitness, and stress management. Intermingled with these programs are efforts aimed at sustaining participation. Finally, environmental changes that support positive health practices are engineered by the *Live for Life* program management team.

The results of the *Live for Life* program have been examined within the context of a rigorous epidemiological evaluation. Preliminary evidence clearly suggests that employees in the treatment cohort, in comparison with controls, consistently show greater improvements in the major health and life-style areas addressed by the *Live for Life* program. Similarly, participation data strongly suggest that the *Live for Life* program process is capable of achieving high and sustained involvement among employees. An economic analysis is currently in progress to estimate the cost–benefit of the *Live for Life* program.

The ultimate judges of program's effectiveness are the management and employees of Johnson & Johnson. The *Live for Life* program must constantly satisfy the health enhancement needs of this diverse customer base. This is the most fundamental law of marketing. Although the preliminary evidence from the *Live for Life* program epidemiological study suggests that customer response has been extremely positive, careful attention to customer needs must be maintained if the *Live for Life* program is to prosper over time.

Acknowledgment

The basic marketing concepts presented here were originally developed by Gene E. Hollen and John H. Rassweiler.

REFERENCES

Campbell, D. T., & Stanley, J. C. *Experimental and quasi-experimental designs for research.* Chicago: Rand-McNally College Publishing Company, 1963.

Cook, T. D., & Campbell, D. T. The design and conduct of quasi-experiments and true experiments in field settings. In M. D. Dunnette (Ed.), *Handbook of industrial and organization psychology.* Chicago: Rand-McNally and Company, 1976.

8

Health Marketing in a Hospital Setting

The Behavioral Medicine Clinic

JOHN E. MARTIN and DONALD M. PRUE

THE PROBLEM

In recent years, there has been a proliferation of research indicating that the main health problems in the United States today are chronic diseases of regulation, such as coronary heart disease and hypertension, which may be prevented or improved through behavioral treatment of risk factors (e.g., smoking treatment). Partly in response to this growing body of epidemiological and treatment research (Levy & Moskowitz, 1982; Matarazzo & Carmody, 1982; Pomerleau & Brady, 1979) a greater number of medical centers are now acknowledging the need for behavioral medicine services within the confines of the hospital.

Two additional factors have facilitated the utilization of behavioral medicine programs by hospitals. First, the roots of the behavioral medicine clinic are embedded deeply in the training hospitals of our medical schools. Much of the pioneering work in the areas of biofeedback and behaviorally based treatment on coronary heart disease, hypertension, pain, stress-related disorders, obesity, and smoking has been conducted and refined at medical schools, particularly in the United States (Miller, 1981; Pomerleau & Brady, 1979; Williams & Gentry, 1977). Second, over the past 10 to 15 years, these experimental programs have often evolved to the point where they are considered a clinical service even in the nonresearch/nontraining hospital.

JOHN E. MARTIN and DONALD M. PRUE • Veterans Administration Medical Center, Jackson, Mississippi 39216. This research and chapter preparation were supported in part by the Medical Research Service of the Veterans Administration Grant Nos. 4187-002, 4187-003, and 9865-001.

For example, even 5 years ago, a hospital rarely had biofeedback capabilities, stress management, or even alcohol treatment programs. Yet, today these clinics are much more common.

Although some of the earlier biofeedback and psychosomatic disorders clinics within the medical center have indeed broadened in scope to include more comprehensive treatment of high risk behaviors for disease (Weiss, Heard, & Fox, 1979) and unhealthy life-style (Farquhar, 1979), the overall numbers still seem disappointingly low. It is clear that the initial establishment and subsequent effective operation of these behavioral medicine hospital clinics can be a highly complex and very problematic venture. Perhaps the most important oversight by those responsible for implementing these clinics is with respect to the selling or marketing of the programs to the patient consumers and hospital staff alike. In particular, failure to attend to the principles and procedures of effective marketing may account for the relatively few behavioral medicine programs accepted and fully utilized in hospitals today.

This chapter describes our efforts to develop health services and to effectively market several behavioral medicine programs at the Jackson, Mississippi, Veterans Administration (VA) Medical Center. A market analysis will be described, including our early attempts to implement a headache/pain clinic and a stress management program, followed by a step-by-step look at the smoking and the hypertension education programs. These latter case examples will also include a cost-efficiency analysis to illustrate a relatively simple procedure for more objectively evaluating the efficiency of the marketing strategies. Our emphasis will be on the relative effectiveness and efficiency of various marketing strategies, including product promotion and manipulations of product packaging and program placement that affected utilization of our services. It is hoped that our experience, as described here, will aid others in establishing or furthering the impact of behavioral medicine programs within their own hospital settings.

MARKET ANALYSIS

One could easily assume, as we initially did, that the provision of behavioral medicine and health improvement services within the hospital would simply consist of informing referral agents and patients of the health service. Presumably health programs such as those concerned with pain and stress management, smoking treatment and cardiovascular health education respresent highly desirable *products*. If these services are then offered at a favorable *price* and are situated in a good *place,* little else should be required for the rapid acceptance and utilization of the programs. It was not quite so simple. A number of important problems and inhibiting factors greatly reduced our initial effectiveness in implementing the programs and attracting a steady flow of patients.

Our initial market analysis consisted of surveying various hospital staff and patients and of compiling our own early experiences subsequent to implementing two clinics in the medical center—the Headache/Pain Clinic and the Stress Management Clinic. Our survey and early experience indicated that there were at least four major stumbling blocks to the initiation of behavioral medicine programs.

First of all, our 500-bed medical/training hospital, like most others, was established on a disease model of service delivery, a model that has important implications for the establishment and utilization of behavioral medicine programs. The *disease model* implicitly assumes that the best approach to health (in this case nondisease) is the attenuation of symptoms or complaints. The patient comes to the hospital with the expectation of being effectively treated (that is, cured), whereas the medical staff's expectations primarily involve the alleviation of symptoms and, if possible, the effective control of the disease. This approach and a goal of nondisease leads hospitals to neglect health as an important organizational mission. Hospital procedures established within this framework generally fail to consider the growing body of research indicating that behavioral factors are often the principal risk factors for a variety of chronic diseases. For example, the cardiovascular diseases such as coronary heart disease (CHD), hypertension, and atherosclerosis are by far the leading causes of morbidity and mortality in the industrialized world today (Levy & Moskowitz, 1982). Significantly, the primary risk factors for these disease processes are essentially *behavioral.* They include smoking, poor eating, stress management habits, and physical inactivity. Yet, much hospital care is now devoted to the tertiary care of patients with cardiovascular disease and its sequelae, with little or no attention devoted to the modification of behavioral risk factors.

Second, when physicians, nurses, and other hospital staff members do consider the importance of behavioral risk factors, their own technology, consisting of invasive, physiological, or pharmacological procedures, has very little impact on modifying these behaviors. Not surprisingly, verbal admonishment, which is their principal strategy, has fared poorly. This failure, in turn, decreases the likelihood that future efforts will be made to target and change relevant health behaviors by the medical staff. Perhaps the best example of this situation is the problem of cigarette smoking. Physicians' advice to their patients to stop smoking has typically had a low success rate (Russell, Wilson, Taylor, & Baker, 1979). Although this practice might be good from an overall public health standpoint, on a more personal level it is understandably difficult for the physician to persist in admonishing smoking patients when this strategy is generally unsuccessful. Further, and perhaps more importantly, it then may become easy to lose sight of the fact that there might be other things that can be done for patients who do not respond to verbal admonishment alone.

Third, programs directed at issues of health and the reduction of risk have only recently been developed. Programs have been largely experimental, and success rates have been quite variable. In fact, for many problems, treatment of proven efficacy has yet to be developed. The fact that this volume is only now being published suggests that there has not been a concerted effort to promote health-oriented programs for widespread adoption in health service systems. Thus, routine referral to health-oriented programs has not become an established medical center procedure largely because these programs have not been available heretofore.

Finally, even in areas of more proven efficacy, behavioral medicine programs may have been underutilized because of their association with psychology and psychiatry. Because these professions are identified with the treatment of mental illness, patients and medical center professionals may be reluctant to consider seeking services unless there are obvious psychological problems. The stigma attached to seeing a psychologist or other mental health professional may prevent physician referrals as well as patient-initiated contacts for the newer services of the behavioral medicine psychologist.

It appeared, then, that the limited awareness and utilization of behavioral medicine programs within our medical center could be attributed in large part to the four inhibiting factors noted: (1) the medical model emphasis on treatment of overt disease; (2) the failure of medical professionals to acknowledge the existence of behavioral techniques for modifying disease risk factors; (3) the relative unavailability of effective behavioral medicine programs; and (4) the stigma attached to seeing a psychologist. In our opinion, these factors constituted ever-present and formidable hurdles that required intense, and perhaps continual, marketing interventions. In addition to these major constraints, there were a number of other important stumbling blocks to successfully establishing behavioral medicine at the Jackson VA Medical Center. These were discovered through our attempts to pilot two clinics—stress management and headache/pain. These other problems are detailed in the following section.

Headache/Stress Management Programs

An overall analysis of the marketing environment in the hospital was conducted within the context of a pilot implementation of a headache program and a stress management program for patients and staff. The Jackson VA headache/pain and stress management programs were the first behavioral medicine programs systematically implemented in the hospital, beginning around 1976–1977. The programs were the result of behavioral medicine staff interest in these problems and, in part, due to the high incidence rates in the population of veterans seeking hospital treatment. In addition, hospital personnel occasionally requested consultation in these areas for individual patients presenting with intractable complaints. However, the low frequency of the referrals prevented cost-efficient, group treatment of these problems. Prior to developing our marketing strategy, which will be detailed later, patients were seen in individual therapy—a treatment arrangement that was less desirable than group treatment.

The Headache/Pain Clinic and Stress Management Clinic were originally promoted through announcements at hospital staff and ward meetings. Yet, this apparently logical first step was unsuccessful in substantially increasing referrals to these programs. Several brainstorming sessions suggested that the problem might lie in the referral process and low staff and patient awareness of our programs. Particularly problematic in this regard was the large turnover in residents and medical students who rotated through our medical center. Informal questioning of hospital staff indicated that relatively few medical staff were aware of the existence of the clinics at all, let alone being aware of who was eligible and the formal mechanisms of referral. There was an obvious need to make medical staff continuously aware of the operation of these new programs using methods other than the staff education procedure devised initially. As a result of this situation, we decided to take the unprecedented step within our medical complex of advertising our programs in the physician and direct care areas of the hospital.

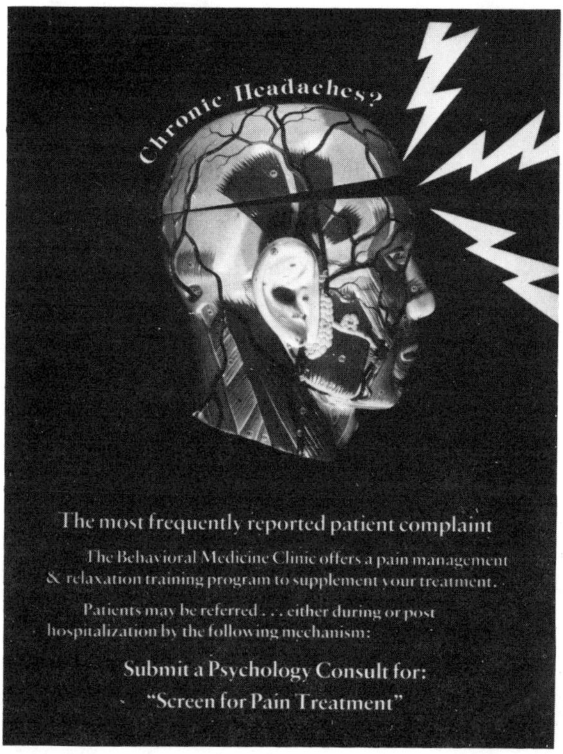

Figure 1. Headache/pain poster employed in promoting the pain program throughout the medical center.

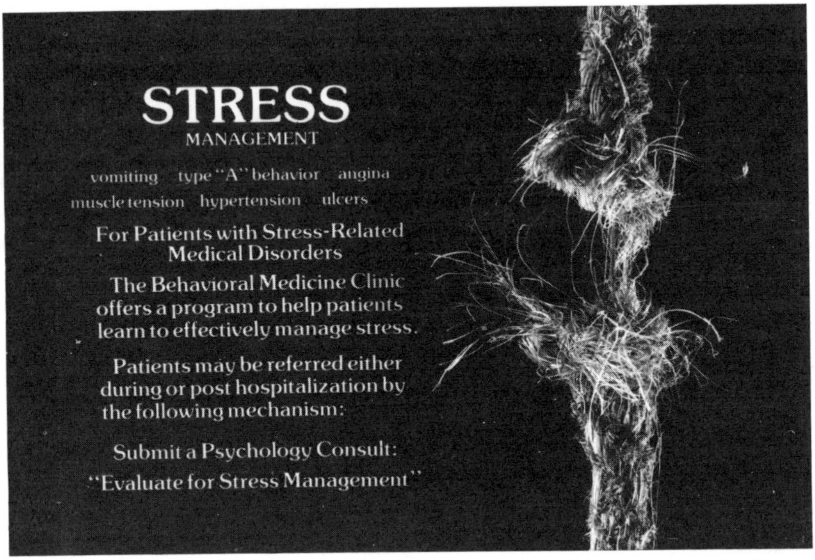
STRESS
MANAGEMENT
vomiting type "A" behavior angina
muscle tension hypertension ulcers
For Patients with Stress-Related Medical Disorders
The Behavioral Medicine Clinic offers a program to help patients learn to effectively manage stress.
Patients may be referred either during or post hospitalization by the following mechanism:
Submit a Psychology Consult: "Evaluate for Stress Management"

Figure 2. Stress management poster employed in promoting the stress management program throughout the medical center.

The behavioral medicine program staff, in conjunction with the Medical Media Service, developed a series of attractive posters designed to illustrate the headache/pain and stress management programs. These posters were prominently displayed in areas of the hospital frequented by physicians and medical staff. Figures 1 and 2 show the (29 cm × 38 cm) posters. Evaluation of the effects of this intervention indicated that referrals doubled within 2–4 weeks. However, the referral rate decreased after 4–6 weeks at the higher rate.

Because of the relatively positive response to the headache and stress management posters, it was decided to employ similar procedures systematically in marketing the two newer programs that were being developed by behavioral medicine. The Smoking Treatment and Research Clinic and the Hypertension Patient Education Program were targeted at this point, and a more formal marketing program was developed and implemented for each. These two marketing efforts will now be described in some detail.

CASE EXAMPLE 1: THE SMOKING TREATMENT PROGRAM

Market Analysis

Given the high frequency of headache and stress problems, it was not difficult to establish the need for our treatment programs within the medical center. Yet, a more important medical problem—smoking—had been virtually neglected by medical and behavioral medicine staff. This was somewhat surprising because the World Health Organization has targeted smoking as the most important preventable health risk in the industrialized world today. Smoking has been causally linked to a variety of cancers, lung disease, and most importantly, cardiovascular disease; the latter is responsible for over half of all deaths among Americans (Levy & Moskowitz, 1982). In short, smoking treatment is especially critical within a medical center that is devoted to treating mostly smoking-related disorders. Further, in our particular hospital, one survey indicated that roughly 90% of all the inpatients and a considerable proportion of the staff were smokers. This exceptionally high percentage of patient smokers may be fairly representative of our VA hospitals that serve many of our older, less healthy veterans. Unfortunately, smokers are notoriously resistant to change (Leventhal & Cleary, 1982). In addition, less than 10% of smokers reported that they would attend clinic programs despite the fact that 90% stated that they would like to quit (Gallup, 1974).

Product, Place, and Price

The *product,* smoking treatment, was provided as a research program to evaluate alternative methods of assessing and treating smoking behavior and overall health risk due to smoking. Both patients and staff were eligible for treatment. The clinic was originally funded through the VA Merit Review Program and was subsequently refunded for an additional 3 years. The overall assessment and treatment procedures are described in greater detail in the section called *treatment interventions.*

The *place* or location of the clinic, although not ideal, was reasonably good. Space for the clinic was allotted by the psychology department and included a rather spartan three-room suite off the fourth-floor elevator lobby, between the Psychology Service, Mental Hygiene Clinic, and the Psychiatry and Internal Medicine Wards. Traffic passing by the clinic was moderate, principally consisting of psychology/psychiatry staff, inpatients and their families, and psychiatry outpatients. Although a considerable proportion of the hospital staff and patients on other floors seldom traveled to the fourth floor, those who did had difficulty missing the clinic. Importantly, the clinic door opened into the fourth-floor elevator lobby, just a short trip up the elevators or stairs from the main lobby.

Finally, the *price,* at least in monetary terms, was unbeatable. Smoking treatment was provided free to veterans and hospital staff. Although the price was considered advantageous, the nonmonetary (psychic) costs to consumers were considered potentially very high. For example, the pain of psychological and physical withdrawal from tobacco is generally well known among smokers, not to mention the considerable response cost involved in attending numerous assessment and treatment sessions, self-monitoring requirements, intensive behavior modification techniques, and dealing with powerful urges to smoke. One further concern was the fact that this cost had to compete with our own hospital canteen store that sold cigarettes at well below retail prices.

Unfortunately, a highly desirable product, relatively favorable price, a fairly good location, and considerable word-of-mouth announcing the clinic's opening were insufficient in stimulating a significant number of smoker referrals. The need for more powerful, systematic marketing efforts became very apparent at this point.

The Marketing Program

Over the course of the next 14 months, various marketing strategies were evaluated with respect to the number of referrals to the smoking clinic during each marketing intervention. Each intervention was continued for a minimum of 4 weeks and until relative stability in referral rate occurred.

Eight different marketing/promotional interventions were employed within a 14-month period. These marketing treatments were at times combined, or withdrawn, to determine the specific effects of each. The irreversible, historical effects of each intervention on subsequent intervention periods did, however, make it impossible to isolate their independent effects completely.

The marketing of the smoking program within the hospital consisted of various promotional campaigns, changes in program accessibility (place), and finally, modifications in the treatment response cost (price) through changes in the treatment procedures (product). The patient and staff consumers and the medical staff referral agents were all considered important to the effective marketing of the program.

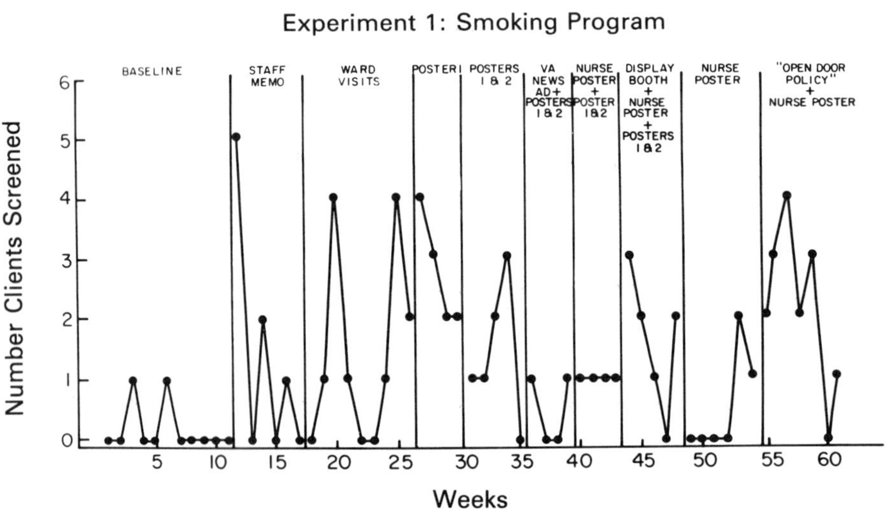

Figure 3. Number of smoking clients screened for treatment. The data points represent the total number of smokers screened per week, across 61 weeks and various marketing interventions.

Therefore, interventions were aimed at the three groups, together or individually. The promotional efforts included announcements of the program at staff meetings throughout the hospital, a memorandum sent to all physicians and wards, personal visits to wards to recruit smokers, posters advertising the program placed around the hospital, a staff newspaper advertisement, and a special display booth.

An attempt was also made to improve referral rates through changes in the placement of the program by increasing access to the clinic. Finally, special attention was given to the problem of the considerable effort or response cost required of the smoking client. The assessment and treatment procedures were streamlined to minimize the reluctance of smokers to come to the clinic, decrease dropouts, and increase program satisfaction. These changes were intended to maximize word-of-mouth referrals from pleased customers to smoker friends and acquaintances.

RESULTS

Promotional Interventions

Clinic Announcements (Word-of-Mouth Baseline)

During the initial 11 weeks, the opening and purpose of the smoking clinic was announced by psychology personnel at hospital staff meetings, administrative meetings, and ward staffings throughout the hospital. Figure 3 shows the effect on referral rate of the initial announcements. These announcements had very little impact on referrals, with only two formal referrals occurring in the 11-week period. Analysis of the type of referral, self or staff (Figure 4), indicated no differences. We were initially surprised over the general absence of referrals. When it became obvious that this informal promotion of the clinic was clearly not the way to increase referrals, we employed the more formal strategy of a medical center memorandum.

Memorandum to All Physicians and Wards

After discontinuation of the ineffective verbal announcements, a formal memorandum was sent to staff physicians, interns, and residents as well as to all wards in the hospital. The memo announced the smoking treatment clinic, its location, procedures, targeted clients, and mechanisms for referral. Another memorandum was devised for patients and distributed on wards and patient areas. As indicated by Figure 3, this resulted in a considerable increase in referrals, primarily in the first week. However, a significant downward trend in referrals was apparent after the first week. The increase in referrals was accounted for mostly by staff members referring patients, for example, a physician or nurse sending a consult form on a smoking patient (Figure 4).

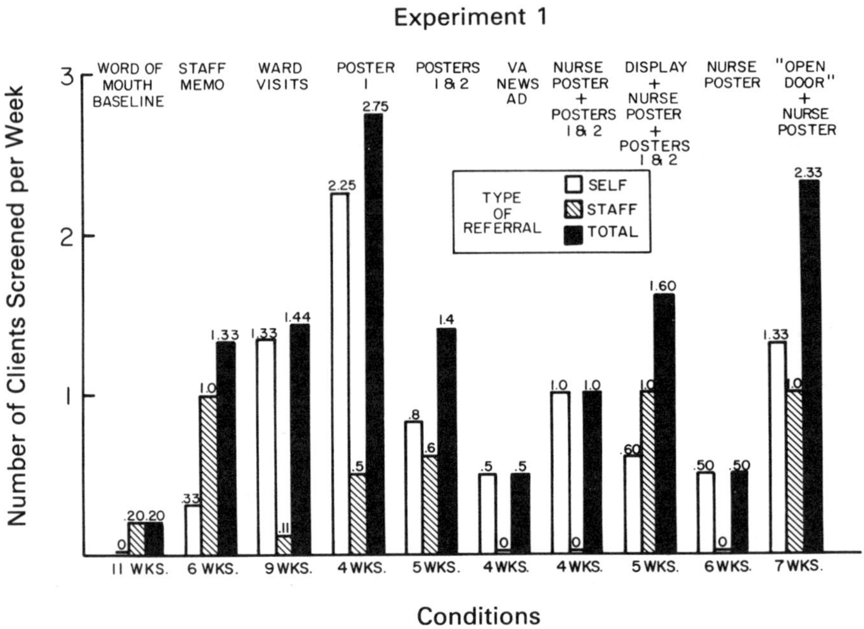

Figure 4. Number of smoking clients screened for treatment by referral type. Total, self- and staff referrals are shown for each condition.

Ward Visits

The third intervention was a more powerful, but costly, one. It consisted of visits to all wards to announce the smoking clinic and to prompt referrals from ward physicians and nurses. In this intervention, smoking clinic staff personally visited each patient ward in the hospital on a weekly basis. During these visits, at least one physician *and* one nurse were consulted to describe the program and referral process. Medical staff were encouraged to talk to other staff and patients regarding the clinic. Smoking program staff were instructed to speak to different physicians and nurses on individual wards at subsequent weekly visits. Compared to the memorandum, ward visits and prompts had a similar but more consistent effect on total referrals (Figure 3). This increase was accounted for by a considerable increase in self-referrals (Figure 4). Interestingly, the net result of the intervention was that staff came for treatment rather than referring more patients.

Following this 9-week phase, the next logical step to recruit patients seemed to be to contact the patients even more directly. Because talking to each patient individually was deemed impractical, a more efficient, mass marketing intervention was implemented using poster advertisements in patient areas of the hospital.

Posters

The fourth strategy consisted of displaying smoking program posters (29 cm × 38 cm) in patient areas, wards, cafeterias, admissions and outpatient areas, waiting rooms, and high-traffic lobbies of the hospital. The posters were developed by the smoking clinic staff and the hospital's medical media department and are shown in Figures 5 and 6.

The effects of the two posters were evaluated, in additive fashion, such that Poster 1 (Figure 5) was first displayed and then Poster 2 (Figure 6) was added. Twenty posters were distributed to various patient and visitor areas in each of the two poster conditions.

Results of the Poster 1 condition indicated that its display around the hospital was associated with a considerable, though variable, volume of referrals (Figure 3). Significantly, this referral rate (11) represented an amount approximately equal to that stimulated by ward visits (13) but in less than half the time (4 weeks vs. 9

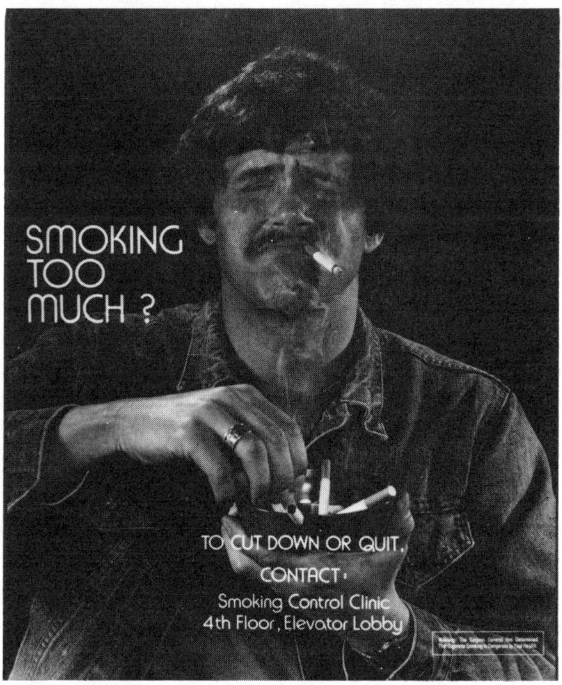
SMOKING
TOO
MUCH ?
TO CUT DOWN OR QUIT,
CONTACT:
Smoking Control Clinic
4th Floor, Elevator Lobby

Figure 5. Smoking program Poster 1. This poster was initially displayed within the medical center to promote smoker referrals to the clinic. (This particular poster was an award-winning poster at a national medical media conference.)

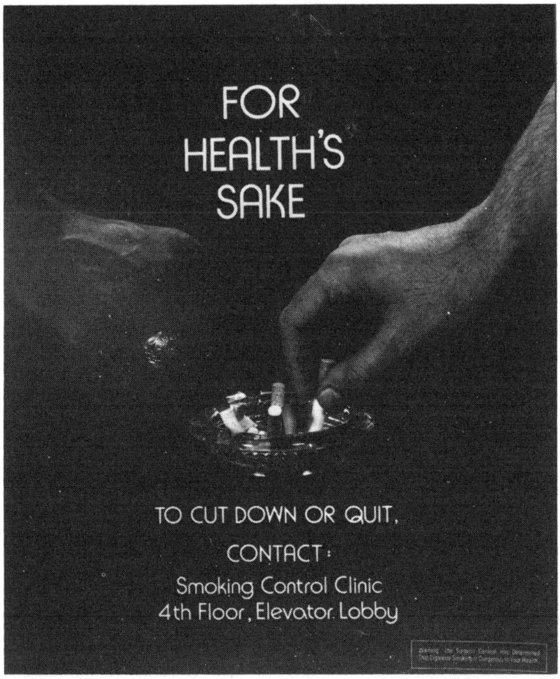
FOR
HEALTH'S
SAKE
TO CUT DOWN OR QUIT,
CONTACT:
Smoking Control Clinic
4th Floor, Elevator Lobby

Figure 6. Smoking program Poster 2. This poster was subsequently displayed with Poster 1 to promote smoker referrals throughout the medical center.

weeks). This increase in referrals was a function of increases in staff and self-referrals (Figure 4). More importantly, the self-referrals were patients rather than staff members.

Addition of the second poster, the Poster 1 and 2 condition, was associated with a somewhat surprising decrease in overall referrals in the first 2 weeks. This was followed by an increase in referrals over the second 2 weeks and a precipitous drop in the fifth and final week of the intervention. Rate of self-referrals decreased by roughly two thirds whereas staff referrals increased an average of .1 per week (Figure 4). Several explanations were offered for this reduction. First, the more or less steadily decreasing referral rate from the first week of the Poster 1 condition (Figure 3) suggested a possible novelty effect of the poster placement followed by habituation to the posters. That is, people noticed and perhaps remembered the posters when they were first displayed but gradually habituated to their presence. Second, it is possible that Poster 2 was a less eye-catching poster, thereby diluting the message. The decline in referrals led to continued efforts to recruit smokers. Following the fifth week of the Poster 1 and 2 condition, an ad was placed in the VA employees' newsletter.

Staff Newspaper Advertisement

An advertisement containing information similar to that in the original staff memo was placed in the *VA News,* a monthly publication routinely sent to all professional and nonprofessional staff of the VA medical center. The posters were left up during this condition. As illustrated in Figures 3 and 4, overall rate of self- and staff referrals dropped considerably. The continued drop in referrals was not affected by the *VA News* ad, suggesting that it had little or no independent effect on smoker referrals. At this point, we hypothesized that a more focused effort directed to the nursing staff might result in more referrals.

Nurse Posters Plus General Hospital Posters

During the next 4-week period, an additional poster was placed on a prominent wall in each ward nurses' station in the medical center. Permission was requested of each head nurse before hanging the posters. At the same time, the head nurse was encouraged to use the poster as a cue to inform other staff and patients about the smoking clinic. Other posters around the hospital were retained as originally positioned in the Poster 1 and 2 conditions. Results of the nurses' station poster placement suggested only a slight improvement in overall referral rate (Figure 3) with a twofold increase in self-referrals accounting for this increase (Figure 4).

The Check-Your-Smoking-Health-Risk Display Booth

Because of the problems in attracting clients to the smoking clinic, an attempt was made to take the clinic to the potential clients. Referrals were tracked for 5 weeks following the placement of a 1-day smoking display booth in the first floor main lobby of the medical center. The booth was staffed throughout the day with at least two smoking-clinic personnel. The purpose of the booth was to provide information about the clinic—written materials describing the smoking clinic and the mechanism of entry were provided—and to assess carbon monoxide (CO) levels of interested smokers. Carbon monoxide measurement was used by the clinic for several reasons. First, CO is considered the most important of the poisonous gases in tobacco smoke due to its association with cardiovascular disease in smokers (Frederiksen & Martin, 1979). Second, it is easily and reliably measured. Smokers blow up a small bag that is then connected to an analyzer that provides a CO level in about 15 seconds (Hughes, Frederiksen, & Frazier, 1978). Finally, smokers report that they particularly like the CO feedback about their health risk level (Martin & Frederiksen, 1980)—an attraction that was apparently not restricted to smokers in the clinic.

The display booth was a popular success. Over 300 smokers had their CO level checked during the day. As shown in Figures 3 and 4, the addition of the 1-day booth accounted for a 60% increase in overall referrals. The majority occurred in the first 2 weeks of this condition. Yet, the CO booth was also followed by progressively fewer referrals across weeks. Given the 1-day nature of the intervention, this trend is not too surprising. The results suggest the short-term impact of brief promotional displays both on health consumer and referral agent behavior. Curiously, the display booth was associated with 40% decrease in smoker self-referrals (Figure 4). The overall increase in referrals was accounted for by a 100% increase in staff referrals of smokers.

The results of this intervention further accentuated the short-term effectiveness of this type of strategy. However, it should be noted that the clinic booth was responsible for some smokers coming to the clinic up to 6 months later. These individuals typically stated that their CO had been upsettingly high and that it had taken some time to finally decide to consult the clinic.

Nurse Posters Only

This 6-week intervention was originally intended to be a complete withdrawal of the promotional procedures and materials (e.g., posters) to check for maintenance in the absence of posters. As often happens in this type of clinical research, an oversight occurred: Some of the posters in the nurses' station were inadvertently left in place. Results depicted in Figures 3 and 4 suggest that the condition was associated with a considerable drop in overall referrals and a cessation of staff referrals. Thus, in spite of a number of the nurse posters remaining up, this had apparently ceased to influence their referring behavior.

Program Location/Accessability Interventions

Open-Door Policy

The final 7-week intervention consisted of a simple but apparently very important change in physical access to the program. Because the smoking clinic door opened into the elevator lobby, the door had been kept closed to reduce noise and other distractions. It was decided to evaluate the effect of leaving the door open throughout the working day. Figure 3 illustrates the increase in overall smoker referrals associated with the "open-door policy." This simple easing of program access resulted in another important upturn in smokers' entry into the clinic. Predictably, the major portion of this increase consisted of self-referred walk-ins (Figure 4).

In general, the promotional interventions stimulated both self- and staff referrals of smokers to the clinic. The success of each strategy varied, although all seemed to have one commonality. Whatever the effect on referrals, it was only temporary. This not only suggested to us the importance of varying our promotions and not sticking with a single one for too long a period but also the importance of having a *product* that would "sell" over the mid and long term through its own excellent reputation. It was at this point that we turned our attention from the promotional to the qualitative aspects of our product—the smoking treatment itself.

Treatment Product and Price Interventions

Analysis

During the very early stages of the program, few individuals came to the smoking clinic because they had heard positive things about our program. This situation may have been related to a disturbingly high initial drop-out rate: Over 75% of those accepted for treatment dropped out before the end of treatment. We attributed this high dropout rate to the large catchment area of almost 400 miles in diameter for our medical canter. Thus, patients often had to drive long distances to return for treatment. The combination of a high dropout rate and the apparent failure of smoking treatment clients to recommend the program to other smokers led to close examination of our clinic practices. This, in turn, was followed by a systematic restructuring of our assessment and treatment procedures to suit the special requirements of the veteran seen in our medical center better.

The main theme of our program changes was to minimize the amount of effort required of smokers while simultaneously enhancing the overall effectiveness of treatment. We had determined that our program, although provided at no financial cost to the client, had a very high initial effort cost to the smoker. The high effort was associated with a lengthy assessment regimen that included a 1–2 hr detailed smoking history interview, biochemical testing, paper-and-pencil questionnaires, and a 1–2-week intensive self-monitoring period in which smokers recorded detailed information on smoking antecedents, consequences, and rate. This assessment was then followed by 2 hr of smoking education, highlighting the causes, medical dangers, and benefits of smoking cessation. Finally, six weekly, 1–1½-hr group treatment sessions were conducted. Smokers continued to self-monitor, and they followed a standard behavioral cessation regimen. Treatment included contracting and stimulus control procedures, relaxation training, substance change, rate reduction, and urge control. We acknowledged that this standard behavioral approach to smoking treatment did represent a moderately complex and demanding program. Consequently, we had a difficult time keeping smokers in assessment, much less in treatment.

Low Ball

Based on the preceding analysis, we redesigned the assessment and treatment components to minimize the front-end requirements of each. In this way, smokers hearing about the minimal requirements of the program would be more likely to agree to at least attempt the program. This initial commitment would be followed by success at the early stages and gradually increasing (i.e., low-balling) requirements toward the middle and end of the treatment period. Once the client became committed to the therapy and successfully completed early steps in treatment, then more complex and demanding treatment procedures would be introduced. At that point, the client would likely be more willing to attempt the high-effort requirements of treatment and less willing to waste prior effort expended in treatment. To provide an analogy from sales and marketing literature, a consumer comes to purchase the bargain item and ends up buying other products, even though the overall cost is considerably more than was initially bargained for.

Product (Clinic) Modifications

The first modification was to reduce the initial screening and assessment. Screening was reduced from a 3-hr assessment and 1 week of intensive self-monitoring to a single, 30-min session. The session included biochemical tests of smoking exposure and related health risk and a greatly abbreviated smoking-history questionnaire. The latter was obtained by clinic staff during an interview to increase personal contact. Formerly, the history form was completed by patients. We also decided to look at the self-monitoring component of assessment and treatment because research with similar populations of smokers (Moss, Prue, Lomax, & Martin, 1982) indicated that the greater the self-monitoring requirements the higher the dropout. As the reader will recall, we asked our smokers to record much information—time of cigarette, setting, others present, feelings, and cigarette enjoyment—almost throughout the assessment and treatment period. We reduced the recording requirements to monitoring smoking rate only and the monitoring period to 1 week. Objective measures of tobacco exposure such as CO were used to supplement this information.

Treatment was begun after the 1-week baseline period and included two phases. Phase I was termed *brand fading* and consisted of gradual reductions in tar and nicotine content of the substance smoked through progressive brand changes (Prue, Krapfl, & Martin, 1981). This phase lasted between 4 and 12 weeks. The treatment was designed to require very little of the smoker. The client was not required to reduce smoking rate, only to change to brands lower in tar and nicotine approximately every 2 weeks. Smokers reported that it was very easy to make these changes. When clients reached an ultralow-tar-and-nicotine substance ($<.2$ mg nicotine), they were then offered the option of Phase 2, or cessation training. Phase 2 consisted of a 4-week behavioral smoking cessation package. However, the components of this phase were simpler than those in our earlier cessation program.

Results

Although specific referral data could not be isolated as a function of each of the series of treatment modifications, we did determine that the combined effect of minimizing entry and early assessment/treatment requirements and streamlining treatment was to reduce early treatment dropouts drastically. The program greatly enhanced treatment effectiveness simply because more smokers were completing treatment. The dropout rate was reduced from 75% to 15%. This represented a reduction of 80%. Also, numerous self-referrals reported that they had come because they had heard such positive things about the clinic from others. The net result of our assessment and treatment modifications has been to enhance our clinic marketing efforts greatly, though not to the extent of eliminating the need for continued promotion. This combination of lowering the product cost and improving the overall quality of the product represented perhaps the most important component of our continued success in marketing the smoking program.

A more recent modification of our program has involved the provision of Phases 1 and 2 of brand fading by telephone (Prue, Davis, Martin, & Moss, in press). As noted earlier, the large catchment area of our VA medical center seemed to affect our dropout rates. In addition, a large percentage of smokers were not even accepted for treatment because they did not agree to come to the clinic for weekly treatment sessions. A minimal contact brand-fading treatment program delivered by telephone was devised to improve services to the veteran smokers. The program was piloted on 40 smokers who stated they could not attend clinic sessions. The results indicated that over 75% completed the program and 1-year follow-up contact. We are encouraged by this outcome in light of the fact that these smokers were not treated with our standard in-clinic treatment program. In addition, 25% of the 40 smokers were abstinent at 1-year follow-up. Based on these data, we have subsequently modified our program to treat the majority of referred smokers by telephone.

SMOKING PROGRAM MARKETING: SUMMARY OF RESULTS

The general results of the marketing interventions suggest that staff and patient prompts were effective in producing a 50% to 300% increase in both self- and staff referrals to the clinic over a short period of time. Greater initial effects gave way to decreased effects of promotional strategies over time. This pattern indicates a novelty effect followed by subsequent habituation to the promotional material by both consumers and referral agents.

Modifications in the program location/accessibility and the product itself also produced both tangible and intangible results. Enhancing clinic accessibility through keeping the door open was associated with important increases in referrals, whereas the CO display booth produced more referrals. Finally, streamlining and improving the treatment regimen resulted in even more important and long-lasting benefits.

The simplicity and low cost of some of the interventions suggested an additional important measure of the overall effectiveness of promotional strategies—relative cost efficiency. The following section describes an analysis of the relative cost per referral of each of the interventions.

Cost Efficiency

A cost-efficiency analysis was conducted for each intervention to evaluate further their overall utility. Total staff time, salary costs, and materials costs were divided by number of referrals in each condition. The resulting cost per referral figures are shown in Table 1. The key figures shown in Table 1 are the cost to recruit one client (CPC) and the projected cost to recruit 100 clients (CPC_{100}). The formula used for calculation of this latter measure was

$$CPC_{100} = \frac{(A \times B) + (C \times B)}{100}$$

where A = recruitment cost per client (CPC); B = weeks necessary to recruit 100 clients at respective weekly referral rate; and C = staff person's salary costs to continue the promotion. Hence, in the word-of-mouth announcement condition the recruitment cost per client ($16.65) and projected cost to recruit 100 clients ($1,800) were relatively high. The Poster 1 condition compares favorably even with the inherently low-cost memo condition, considering the relatively high initial materials and development costs ($120.00). Although the memo has a lower recruitment cost per client than did the posters ($1.43 vs. $6.71), the picture changes when the efficiency of the interventions in attracting referrals is projected for 100 clients. That is, the cost per client associated with the poster ($181.00) is clearly superior to the memo cost ($277.00) as well as the other conditions. The one exception to this is the open-door condition. The open-door condition represents a different type of intervention because it manipulated accessibility as opposed to promotion. The results of this condition illustrate the significance of seemingly small changes in program characteristics. The modification in the product (treatment programs) was not subjected to a cost-benefit analysis due to the difficulty in documenting the planning time required for the streamlining of the program. However, it is likely that this was a necessary and overall cost-efficient way to reduce dropouts and enhance satisfied customer referrals—a seemingly vital source of maintaining the program. It is clear that the best promotional efforts will doom an inferior product to a quick death in the consumer marketplace!

Table 1. Recruitment Cost per Client for Smoking Program

Condition	Referral rate (#/wk)	CPC ($)	Projected # wks to recruit 100 clients	Projected CPC to recruit 100 clients ($)	CPC 100[a] (Cost per client for 100 clients [$])
Clinic announcements (word-of-mouth baseline)	.2	0	500	0	1800
Staff memo	1.3	1.42	77	.60	277
Ward visits	1.3	11.65	77	11.00	279
Patient posters	2.0	6.71	50	2.77	181
Combined posters	1.0	5.90	100	2.30	361
Display booth & posters	1.6	27.11	63	20.21	231
Open door policy	2.1	.82	48	—[b]	—[b]
Nurse poster	.5	23.56	200	3.71	721

[a]Including staff salary available time.
[b]Cannot be replicated.

CASE EXAMPLE 2: THE HYPERTENSIVE PATIENT EDUCATION PROGRAM

Market Analysis

Next to smoking, one of the most significant health risks in both hospitalized and nonhospitalized individuals is uncontrolled hypertension (Levy & Moskowitz, 1982). In fact, a large proportion of patients in our medical center were admitted for disorders resulting directly or indirectly from uncontrolled hypertension. In the case of hypertension, the most pressing problem, once elevated blood pressure is detected, is ensuring compliance with medical and health regimens required to control blood pressure elevation. Despite the fact that most hypertensives are required to take medication, studies have indicated that 80% fail to take their medication properly and up to 50% do not take it at all (Haynes, Taylor, & Sackett, 1979).

Thus, it was no surprise when our nursing staff voted hypertension as the most important, albeit neglected, patient education area. It was with this mandate that one of the nursing clinical specialists spearheaded an effort to implement an interdisciplinary education program for hypertensives and their families. Nursing, psychology, pharmacy, internal medicine, and dietetics staffs were invited to participate. Psychology staff worked closely on the marketing and evaluation components of this patient education program.

The Product, Place, and Price

The Hypertensive Patient Education Program consisted of a 3-day class for inpatient hypertensives and their families. The complete program consisted of three 1-hr classes held on successive days and repeated each week. Instruction targeted the definition, health risks, and the medical and behavioral control of hypertension. The relationship between personal behavior and hypertension was stressed as was the imporance of patients taking responsibility for controlling their own high blood pressure. In addition, the patients were provided information on VA and community programs for the control of hypertension (e.g., weight modification and stress management clinics, public health clinics). The education program was provided in three 40-min sessions and conducted in one of the visiting rooms on the medicine wards. It was open without charge to all hypertensive patients, their families, and any other interested persons. The 3-day education series was repeated each week. As in the smoking program, a highly desirable product (the nurses, physicians, and especially the hospital administrators were generally highly supportive of the program), a good place, and an excellent price were insufficient to attract a significant number of people to the Hypertensive Patient Education Program.

The Marketing Program

A total of eight promotional strategies and strategy combinations were implemented across the subsequent 12-month period, including announcements at staff meetings, poster advertisements, patient rewards for attendance, staff feedback, praise, and public address (PA) announcements. The effectiveness of each intervention was gauged in terms of the total number of hypertensive patients who attended the program each week. Each intervention was continued for a minimum of 4 weeks. The relative efficacy of the various strategies was evaluated in a manner similar to that used for the smoking clinic. Figure 7 shows the order of strategy implementations and their effects on attendance at the weekly program. The interventions are described in the following section.

Promotional Strategies and Results

Announcements Baseline

Weekly baseline announcements were made concerning the program at the head nurses' meeting. In addition, verbal prompts were given to the nursing staff on the fourth floor medicine wards prior to each class. The nurses were then responsible for delivering nonambulatory hypertensives to the classroom and for locating and sending all appropriate ambulatory hypertensives. This general procedure was followed throughout the entire study. Although we were highly consistent in prompting the medicine ward nursing staff just before each class, the head nurses around the hospital and the nursing staff on the fourth-floor wards were somewhat less consistent in their prompting of other staff and/or patients. In fairness to the nurses, they were often busy with patients and could spare little time to identify and direct patients to our program.

Thus, we were not surprised to learn that only 22 patients attended during the first 4 weeks as a result of our announcements and prompts. Our surveys indicated that there were rarely fewer than 75 hypertensive inpatients and that there were usually considerably more in the hospital at any one time. We were therefore especially concerned to observe the declining trend in referrals, from seven the first week to only two in the fourth week.

Staff Memorandum

A memorandum was then distributed to medical and nursing staff in all wards, clinics, and patient areas. The memo described the program, time, place, targeted patients, and mechanism of referral. As shown in Figure 7, the staff memo had little impact on overall program attendance. In fact, only 15 hypertensives attended the

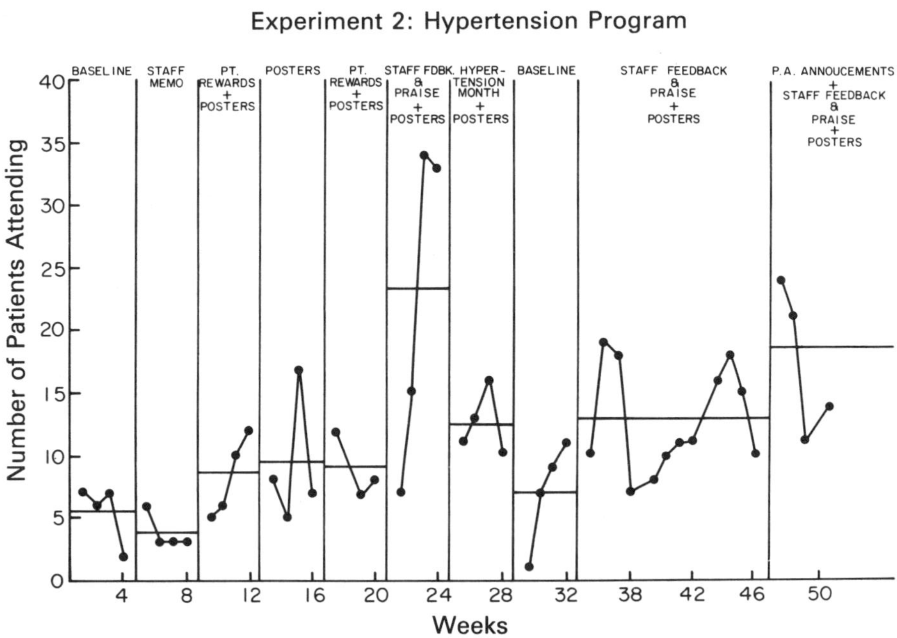

Figure 7. Attendance at Hypertensive Patient Education Program. The data points represent the total number of hypertensive patients attending the program each week. Mean lines are shown for attendance per condition.

program during this second 4-week intervention. Thus, it appeared that the memo added little to the verbal prompting of nurses: The average or mean weekly referral rate was even lower (3.8 per week) than in the initial 4 weeks of verbal prompts (5.5 per week).

Patient Rewards Plus Posters 1

Given the relatively poor results of this type of nurse-focused prompt, it was decided to try a promotional package targeting the hypertensive patients and their families. Figure 8 illustrates one of the posters created to promote the hypertensive patient education program. In addition to the placement of posters in the hospital, patients were rewarded with VA canteen coupon booklets worth $1 each that could be exchanged for goods in the VA canteen store for each session they attended. A brightly colored (7 cm × 12 cm) label announcing the reward for attendance was affixed to each of the posters during the poster-plus-reward condition.

The combined intervention of posters plus reinforcement for attendance was

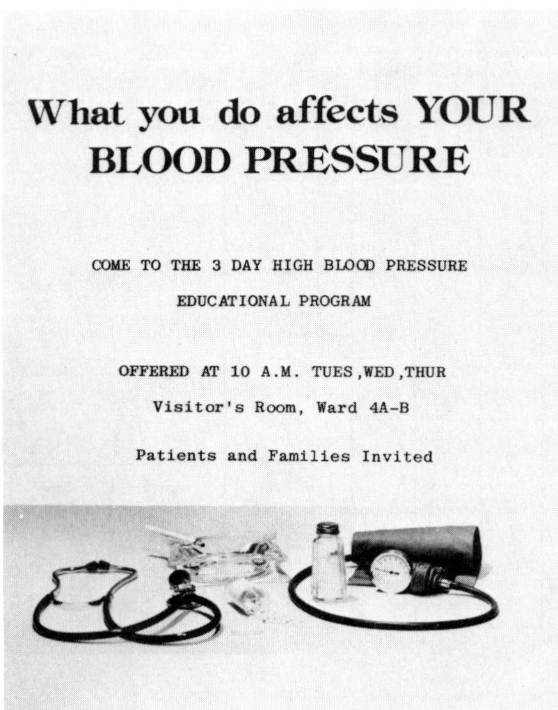

Figure 8. Hypertensive Patient Education Program poster displayed throughout medical center to promote program attendance.

associated with increased attendance. However, we were unsure of which component, the posters or the patient rewards, was responsible for this increase. We withdrew the patient reward because we felt it had not accounted for improved attendance.

Posters Only (Patient Reward Withdrawal)

This intervention was implemented to determine the independent effect of posters on program attendance. In the previous intervention, the majority of patients who attended did not seem interested in the monetary reward. Most had been sent by nurses or had seen the poster. Unfortunately, our attendance data did not distinguish between self-referred or staff-referred hypertensives.

The resulting attendance showed no decrease in attendance as a function of removing the patient reward. In fact, the posters-alone condition was associated with an increase in mean weekly attendance. A replication of the combined intervention was then conducted as a further assessment of the added effect of the monetary reward for attendance.

Patient Reward Plus Posters 2

As is shown in Figure 7, no added effect on program attendance was found for the patient reward. The mean attendance was a slightly lower 9.3 per week.

It had become apparent by this point that many of the patients attending the program had either been told to come or were actually brought to class by the nursing staff. Thus, in a fashion similar to the smoking program marketing, we decided to refocus our attention differently, and much more directly, on the nursing staff.

Staff Feedback and Praise Plus Posters

Two procedures were added to the posters on this intervention. First, whenever a staff member (usually a nurse or nurse's assistant) referred a patient to the program, one of us would personally thank them immediately after class. Second, a graph of program attenders was posted in the head nurses' station on each ward. Each week the total number of hypertensive patients from that ward who attended was plotted on these graphs. Nursing staff were praised for improved or high referral rates. In addition, special recognition was made at weekly head nurses' meetings for improved referral rates and for wards sending the most patients to the program.

The addition of the staff feedback and praise for program referrals was associated with an impressive increase in attendance. Significantly, the peak attendance (34) in the third week was exactly double the previous high (17) in the third week of the poster-alone condition. Further, the increasing attendance rate across the 4 weeks resulted in a mean weekly attendance of 23, almost 2½ times the previous high.

In order to assess the independent effects of the staff feedback and praise procedure further, we planned to discontinue the feedback and praise for a 4-week period. A potential problem with evaluating our promotional efforts developed during the withdrawal of praise and feedback because the experimental condition coincided with National Hypertension Month.

Hypertension Month Plus Posters

Hypertension Month (May) occurred at our medical center in conjunction with the *National High Blood Pressure Education Program*'s High Blood Pressure Awareness Program. It included the presence throughout the month of a blood pressure screening booth in the hospital lobby. In addition, general posters depicting the dangers, detection, and control of high blood pressure were situated throughout the hospital. No systematic effort at promoting the hypertensive patient education class was made during this month. However, hypertensives who had their blood pressure taken at the screeming booth were often informed of the program. Otherwise, the only intervention specific to the class was the presence of program posters in the hospital.

In spite of the hypertension awareness month and its own promotional efforts, our program attendance fell off sharply. That is, the withdrawal of staff feedback and praise was associated with a considerable drop in program attendance. This occurred in spite of the addition of Hypertension Month activities.

Announcement Baseline 2

A return to our original condition was instituted to evaluate the effects of the hypertension booth and posters fully. Figure 7 shows the large reduction in program attendance following the removal of the Hypertension Month booth and the program posters. In the first week of this condition, only one patient attended. This number rose to only 12 in Week 4 (mean = 7 per week). Thus, discontinuation of staff feedback and praise resulted in a 50% drop in referrals, which was followed by an additional 50% decrease after removal of all posters. A final test of the effects of staff feedback and praise and posters combination was then conducted.

Staff Feedback and Praise Plus Posters 2

The procedures in this condition were similar to those used in the first staff-feedback-and-praise-plus-posters condition. The effects were apparent but less profound than during the initial implementation (Figure 7). Peak attendance was 17 in Week 2. Given this somewhat disappointing result, the intervention was repeated for two additional 4-week blocks to test for progressive effects. Yet, as is shown in

Figure 7, the effects across the subsequent 8 weeks were similar to the first 4 weeks (mean = 13 per week). Several explanations for this were ventured, including the possibility that staff may have become satiated by the feedback and praise, and/or they had become habituated to the posters and graphs.

The final strategy was added to the present, moderately effective promotion package in an attempt to overcome any habituation to the posters. The condition employed public address announcements to prompt class attendance. The hospital public address system was chosen because it was inexpensive, reached the entire medical center, appeared underutilized much of the day, and was generally attended to by staff and patients.

Public Address Announcements Plus Ongoing Procedures

This intervention added a brief public address announcement to the ongoing staff-feedback-and-praise-plus-posters condition. The announcement was read by the PA announcer 5–15 min prior to each class. It consisted of an invitation to all hypertensive patients, their families, and interested others to attend the program class.

As is shown in Figure 7, program attendance rose from 11 to 24 in the first week of the added PA announcement. Unfortunately, attendance declined over successive weeks to a level comparable to the prior intervention. Subsequent interventions (not shown) employing only PA announcements were found to be roughly half as effective as the combined-staff-feedback-and-praise-plus-PA-announcements condition. Results of this final intervention strongly suggest that the announcements produced a brief awareness-enhancing effect. This appeared to be followed by a relatively rapid habituation associated with repetitive PA announcements.

HYPERTENSION PROGRAM MARKETING: SUMMARY OF RESULTS

With the exception of the staff memos, all of the prompting procedures (i.e., posters and PA announcements) were effective in stimulating class attendance. Although patient rewards contributed little or nothing to the effectiveness of the poster prompts, interventions directed at the staff were considered to be highly successful. The most effective strategy was providing immediate feedback and praise to nursing staff who referred hypertensive patients to the program. Overall, it was found that the vast majority (87%) of the hypertensive patients were prompted to attend by nurses or nurse assistants.

A number of the interventions lost some effectiveness over time. The same pattern emerged in marketing the smoking program. This seemed to suggest the importance of providing a variety of novel, staff-directed marketing interventions.

One very important aspect of the promotion strategies was their cost in terms of

Table 2. Recruitment Cost per Client (CPC) for Hypertension Program

Condition	Referral rate (#/wk)	CPC ($)	Projected # wks to recruit 100 clients	CPC 100[a] (Cost per client for 100 clients [$])
Announcement baseline	6.3	.79	16	7.96
Staff memo	3.8	2.71	27	14.23
Posters	9.3	2.37	11	6.48
Patient reward plus posters	8.6	2.13	12	7.46
Staff feedback & praise plus posters	14.0	5.10	8	9.57
PA announcements plus staff feedback & praise plus posters	17.5	4.22	6	7.20

[a]Including staff salary classroom time.

human and material resources. The following section provides an analysis of the relative costs of each intervention and gives a more complete picture of the efficiency as well as effectiveness of the interventions.

Cost-Efficiency Analysis

A cost-efficiency analysis was conducted for the hypertension program marketing efforts. The analysis was similar to that conducted for the smoking program. Table 2 provides the recruitment costs per client and per 100 clients across the different conditions. In Table 2, the word-of-mouth baseline resulted in the cheapest CPC ($0.79); however, it would take 16 weeks to recruit 100 clients. This was longer than all other interventions except the memo (27 weeks), costing $7.96 per client when staff salary for class time is considered. The most expensive procedure was the staff feedback and praise with a CPC of $5.10 (highest) and a CPC_{100} of $9.57 (second highest). On the other hand, if speed of obtaining clients is an important consideration, the staff feedback and praise would be the best choice, requiring only 8 weeks to generate 100 clients. Perhaps the most efficient intervention in terms of both cost and potency was the poster intervention. The CPC for the posters was only $2.37; the CPC_{100} was the lowest ($6.48), with just 11 weeks necessary to recruit 100 clients.

SUMMARY AND CONCLUSIONS

This chapter has discussed a number of the problems faced by our behavioral medicine program in implementing health programs within a hospital setting. The chapter described the rationale, procedures, and results of interventions designed to market our programs to hospital staff and patients better. Examples of market analyses, modifications in price, product, place, and promotional strategies have been provided. In addition, anecdotal information and referral and cost-efficiency data have been presented.

Promotional Strategies

Promotional strategies were clearly among the more effective, cheapest, and easiest to implement. Poster-prompting interventions were both effective and highly cost-efficient strategies in recruiting clients to the behavioral medicine programs within the hospital. In fact, follow-up data on the smoking program indicated that almost half of all the clients over a 4-year period came because they saw a poster. Other effective, albeit more costly, interventions were those that incorporated direct contact with the consumer. Direct consumer contact was made during feedback and staff praise, CO booth, and ward visit interventions. Finally, the standard bureaucratic memos and general announcements at staff meetings had little marketing impact.

Our evaluation indicated that the target of the promotional effort determined, to a large degree, whether clients self-initiated referrals or were referred by medical staff. Unfortunately, we did not always target correctly. For example, we felt that patients should assume more responsibility for their health and therefore directed initial promotional efforts to them. It became quite clear, however, that the patient was often a passive recipient of health and medical services. Our data indicate that in some cases our interventions were most successful when directed to *referral* agents. This was particularly true for the hypertensive program: Hypertensive patients (87%) attended because they had been referred by nursing staff. A slightly different picture was found for the smoking program. A 3-year breakdown of how smokers came to the clinic ($N = 243$) revealed that 41% saw the poster, whereas 29% were referred by a physician or nurse. Others came because a friend had recommended it (18%), or they walked by the clinic door (3%). Perhaps the differences across the programs reflected the hypertension program's primary focus on inpatients (roughly 90%).

The focus of promotional campaigns raises important questions as to the desirability of overemphasizing staff referrals. Studies conducted in our medical center (Black, Rothblum, & Massey, 1980) and elsewhere (Goldfried, 1969) have indicated that self-referred patients are less likely to drop out and are more likely to benefit from treatment. This finding presents an interesting dilemma: Should marketing efforts actively target consumers to reach consumers who are then likely to begin and continue a program on their own? Or, should promotions focus on patients via referral agents. As with most either-or dilemmas, the answer probably lies somewhere between the two options. The most pragmatic approach would likely be to target the consumer directly through patient-focused promotions and indirectly through hospital referral-source interventions.

An additional important finding concerns the temporary effectiveness of most promotional interventions. It is possible that patient and staff became habituated or satiated with respect to particular promotion activities much in the same way that they tune out routine announcements over the PA system. A comparable example of this phenomenon was provided by Dawley, Morrison, and Carrol (1980) in their investigation of the effects of no smoking signs within a VA hospital. Dawley *et al.* found that there was some initial compliance when the signs were put up but that this was quickly followed by increasing noncompliance and an eventual return to baseline levels of smoking in those areas of the hospital. A similar habituation would account for referral patterns in our work.

Although somewhat more expensive overall, the direct prompt and feedback interventions did seem to have the most potent effects. Thus, these strategies might be more appropriate for initiating new programs or expanding to new areas of the medical center. The substantial response and time costs could be minimized through switching to a less expensive poster and PA announcement intervention. Routine switching of a variety of promotional activities to highlight the novelty while maintaining "top of the mind awareness" appears to be the best approach for maintaining a high rate of referrals.

Interventions Targeting Place and Product

With respect to the variable of product placement, referral data indicate that minor changes in program location or accessibility can affect referral rates. The open door policy initially made us aware of the importance of access. The recent placement of our smoking clinic in the main traffic artery of the hospital again showed us how important this variable is in initiating novel treatment programs. Again, staff and patients alike are just not accustomed to making referrals outside of well-established hospital services. New programs have to be salient to remain in the consumer's mind to ensure referrals. Product placement can play an important role in attaining program salience.

The product delivered to clients plays an important role in the acceptance of novel programs. Our initial ventures in delivering smoking treatment may provide the best example of the importance of both an effective and reasonably priced product—two aspects that so often compete with one another. We initially developed a very demanding program that required clients to do homework, self-monitor themselves, and make rather dramatic changes in well-learned, albeit bad, habits. The effect of the high response cost was to drive people out of treatment. This problem was exacerbated by the fact that our treatment program was free; therefore there was little monetary incentive to continue treatment.

Our initial reaction to this problem was to blame the victim, smoking veterans, because "everyone knows that behavioral procedures work." Only after a series of product modifications in traditional behavioral procedures (Moss, Prue, Lomax, & Martin, 1982; Prue, Davis, Martin, & Moss, in press), have we been able to approach the success rates of other clinics. Another example of the importance of product changes stemmed from the operation of our headache clinic. During treatment, it became apparent that veterans were not complying with one of the most important components of the program, progressive muscle relaxation (Martin, Collins, Hillenberg, Zabin, & Katell, 1981). Again, a special arrangement had to be made to improve our product so that patients would comply with the procedures. Continued improvements in our products will lead, we hope, to even greater successes with the range of maladaptive or problem behaviors we deal with.

In conclusion, we hope that the information provided in this chapter will be helpful to those readers who are establishing behavioral medicine programs in hospital settings. The information provided might be especially useful to programs that are not consistently attracting a high volume of consumers. As has been illustrated in the immediately preceding pages, effective marketing of health programs must include more than just a concern for the importance of promoting health.

Acknowledgments

The authors wish to acknowledge the instrumental role played by Lee W. Frederiksen in the development and conducting of the marketing campaigns that are described in this chapter. In addition, appreciation is expressed to Jean C. Crawford, R.N., M.S.N., for her extensive collaborative efforts on the development and marketing of the Hypertensive Patient Education Program. The following are also acknowledged for their critical assistance on the smoking and general behavioral medicine marketing interventions: Carol J. Thames and Harriett Fitts Bruno. Finally, we own thanks to Leonard H. Doerfler for his comments on an earlier version of the chapter and to Veola Sherrod, Danley Lomax, and Pamela Childress for their technical assistance.

REFERENCES

Black, J. L., Rothblum, E. D., & Massey, F. H. *The effects of posters in facilitating the implementation of vocational assistance programs.* Unpublished manuscript, 1980.

Dawley, H. H., Jr., Morrison, J., & Carrol, S. Compliance behavior in a hospital setting: Employee and patients' reactions to no-smoking signs. *Addictive Behaviors,* 1980, *5,* 329–331.

Farquhar, J. W. *The American way of life need not be hazardous to your health.* New York: W. W. Norton, 1979.

Frederiksen, L. W., & Martin, J. E. Carbon monoxide and smoking behavior. *Addictive Behaviors,* 1979, *4,* 21–30.

Frederiksen, L. W., Martin, J. E., & Webster, J. S. Assessment of smoking behavior. *Journal of Applied Behavior Analysis,* 1979, *12,* 653–664.

Gallup Poll Index. Report No. 108, June 1974, 20–21.

Goldfried, M. R. Prediction of improvement in an alcoholism outpatient clinic. *Quarterly Journal of Studies on Alcohol,* 1969, *30,* 129–139.

Haynes, R. B., Taylor, D. W., & Sackett, D. L. (Eds.). *Compliance in health care.* Baltimore: Johns Hopkins Press, 1979.

Hughes, J. R., Frederiksen, L. W., & Frazier, M. A carbon monoxide analyzer for measurement of smoking behavior. *Behavior Therapy,* 1978, *9,* 293–296.

Leventhal, H., & Cleary, P. D. The smoking problem: A review of the research and theory in behavioral risk modification. *Psychological Bulletin,* 1982, *88,* 370–405.

Levy, R. I., & Moskowitz, J. Cardiovascular research: Decades of progress, a decade of promise. *Science,* 1982, *217,* 121–129.

Martin, J. E., & Frederiksen, L. W. Self-tracking of carbon monoxide levels by smokers. *Behavior Therapy,* 1980, *11,* 577–587.

Martin, J. E., Collins, F. L., Hillenberg, J. B., Zabin, M. A., & Katell, A. D. Assessing compliance to home relaxation: A simple technology for a critical problem. *Journal of Behavioral Assessment,* 1981, *3,* 193–198.

Matarazzo, J. D., & Carmody, T. P. Health psychology. In M. Hersen & A. S. Bellack (Eds.), *The clinical psychology handbook.* New York: Pergamon, 1982.

Miller, N. E. An overview of behavioral medicine: Opportunities and dangers. In S. Weiss, A. Herd, & B. Fox (Eds.), *Perspectives on behavioral medicine.* New York: Academic Press, 1981.

Moss, R. A., Prue, D. M., Lomax, D., & Martin, J. E. The effects of self-monitored smoking on treatment session attendance. *Addictive Behaviors,* 1982, *7,* 381–385.

Pomerleau, O. F., & Brady, J. P. (Eds.). *Behavioral medicine: Theory and practice.* Baltimore: Williams & Wilkins, 1979.

Prue, D. M., Davis, C. J., Martin, J. E., & Moss, R. A. An investigation of a minimal contact brand fading program for smoking treatment. *Addictive Behaviors,* in press.

Prue, D. M., Krapfl, J. R., & Martin, J. E. Brand fading: The effects of gradual changes to low tar and nicotine cigarette on smoking rate, carbon monoxide and thiocyanate. *Behavior Therapy,* 1981, *12,* 400–416.

Russell, M. A. H., Wilson, C., Taylor, C., & Baker, C. D. Effect of general practitioners' advice against smoking. *British Medical Journal,* 1979, *2,* 231–235.

Weiss, S. M., Heard, J. A., & Fox, B. H. (Eds.). *Perspectives on Behavior Medicine.* New York: Academic Press, 1979.

Williams, R. B. & Gentry, W. D. (Eds.). *Behavioral Approaches to Medical Treatment.* Cambridge, Mass.: Ballinger, 1977.

Index